AFiB

DIET COOKBOOK
FOR BEGINNERS

Simple, Heart-Healthy Recipes to Manage Atrial Fibrillation
and Boost Your Well-Being

Kingsley Klopp

To show our appreciation for your purchase, we're delighted to offer you these special bonuses as a heartfelt thank you

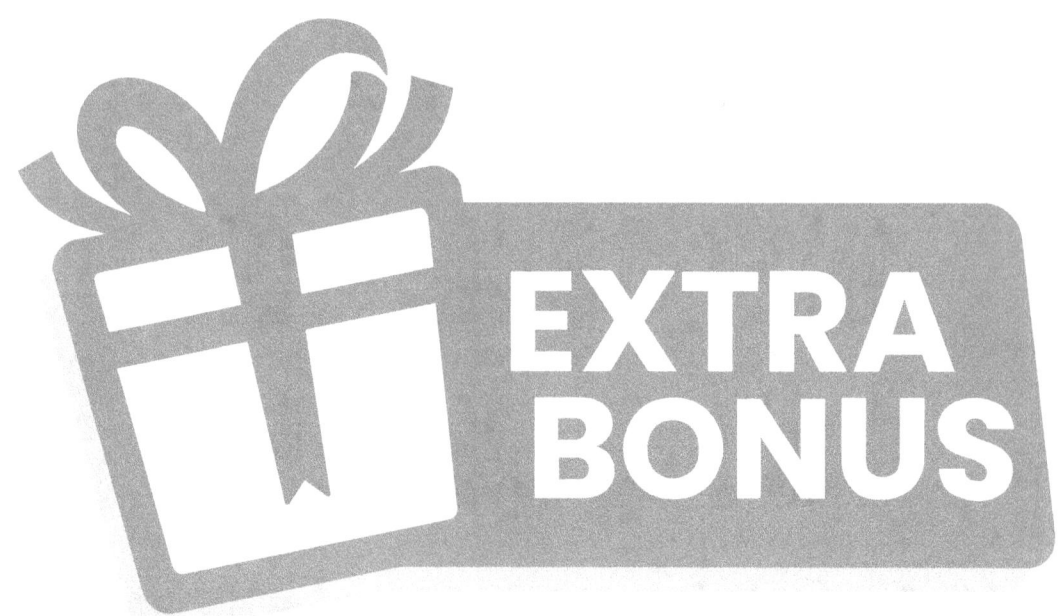

1. A Food Tracker Journal
2. Downloadable E-BOOK featuring full-color images of finished recipes

Table of Content

Introduction...7

Part 1
What is Atrial Fibrillation (AFib)?
- Understanding AFib...9
- Symptoms and Risks...11
- Treatment of AFib...13

Part 2
The AFib Diet Explained
- Importance of Diet in Managing AFib.................................15
- Role of Nutrients and Supplements...................................17

Breakfast Recipes
Apple Cinnamon Oatmeal...20
Banana Nut Oatmeal...21
Berry Oatmeal Smoothie..22
Vegetable Frittata...23
Spinach and Mushroom Omelette...24
Kale and Spinach Smoothie...25
Berry Beet Smoothie..26
Greek Yogurt with Mixed Nuts and Honey...........................27
Pineapple Turmeric Smoothie...27
Berry Parfait...28
Quinoa Breakfast Bowl...28
Whole Wheat Pancakes...29
Barley Porridge...30
Whole Grain Waffles...31
Turkey and Spinach Breakfast Sausages.............................32
Rice Porridge with Berries...33
Sweet Potato Congee..34
Millet Porridge with Apples and Cinnamon..........................35
Buckwheat Porridge with Honey and Walnuts.....................36
Caprese Salad with an Egg...37

Watermelon Salad with Mint and Feta...38
Nutty Granola...39
Seed Mix Topped Yogurt...40
Coconut and Almond Chia Breakfast Bowl...41

Poultry Recipes

Grilled Lemon Herb Chicken...42
Chicken and Vegetable Stir-Fry...43
Baked Chicken with Spinach...44
Chicken Soup with Barley...45
Mediterranean Chicken Salad...46
Chicken Cacciatore...47
Stuffed Chicken Breast...48
Turkey Meatloaf...49
Smoked Turkey Breast...50
Turkey and Quinoa Stuffed Peppers...51
Turkey Bolognese...52
Turkey Skewers with Vegetables...53
Creamy Turkey and Mushroom Soup...54
Chicken and Turkey Sausage Jambalaya...55
Poultry Shepherd's Pie...56
BBQ Pulled Chicken...57
Chicken and Turkey Meatballs...58
Turkey Broth Soup with Kale...59
Turkey Piccata...60
Poached Chicken Salad...61
Turkey and Cranberry Sliders...62
Chicken Paella with Brown Rice...63
Turkey and Spinach Meatballs...64
Turkey Pot Pie...65
Turkey Noodle Soup...66

Fish & Seafood Recipes

Grilled Salmon with Dill...67
Baked Cod with Lemon and Capers...68
Tilapia Piccata...69
Herb-Crusted Halibut...70
Asian-Style Tuna Steaks...71
Poached Salmon with Asparagus...72
Smoked Haddock Chowder...73
Mackerel with Tomato Salad...74
Trout Almondine...75

Shrimp Stir-Fry with Vegetables..76
Garlic Scallops..77
Mussels in Tomato Broth..78
Spicy Shrimp Tacos..79
Scallop and Pea Risotto..80
Seafood Paella..81
Fisherman's Stew..82
Grilled Sea Bass with Mango Salsa..83
Baked Trout with Walnut Crust..84
Cod with Greek Salad..85
Sushi Rolls with Brown Rice..86
Kedgeree with Smoked Fish..87
Fish Fillet with Citrus Quinoa..88
Spicy Tuna Poke Bowl..89
Seafood and Spinach Lasagna..90
Lemon Butter Scampi..91
Baked Catfish with Sweet Potato Fries..92

Soup & Stew Recipes

Japanese Miso-Glazed Cod..93
Carrot Ginger Soup..94
Roasted Butternut Squash Soup..95
Broccoli and Almond Soup..96
Spicy Sweet Potato Soup..97
Cabbage Detox Soup..98
Cream of Mushroom Soup..99
Beetroot and Ginger Soup..100
Chicken Noodle Soup..101
Turkey and White Bean Chili..102
Lentil and Spinach Soup..103
Pea and Ham Soup..104
Beef Barley Soup..105
Italian Meatball Soup..106
Miso Soup with Tofu..107
Egg Drop Soup..108
Moroccan Chickpea Stew..109
Irish Stew with Lamb..110
Beef and Vegetable Stew..111
Brazilian Black Bean Stew..112
Hungarian Mushroom Stew..113
Pork and Tomatillo Stew..114
Spring Vegetable Soup..115

Korean Kimchi Stew..116
Mexican Posole...117
Japanese Ramen..118

Vegetables
Vegetable Lentil Soup..119
Gazpacho..120
Asparagus with Hollandaise Sauce..121
Crispy Zucchini Fritters...122
Eggplant Dip..123
Stuffed Mushrooms..124
Bruschetta with Tomato and Basil...125
Mushroom and Leek Quiche..126
Vegetable Stir Fry with Tofu..127
Grilled Asparagus with Lemon Tarragon Dressing.................................128
Spaghetti Squash with Tomato Sauce...129
Sweet Potato and Black Bean Chill..130
 Zucchini Noodle Salad..131

10-WEEK MEAL PLAN...132

Important Note

We are thrilled to have you join us, and we are committed to making this journey both delicious and beneficial for your well-being. However, before we dive into the recipes, we would like to share a few important notes.

Each individual's dietary needs are unique, especially when managing a condition like AFib. While we have crafted these recipes with heart health in mind, it's essential to remember that your personal health requirements might differ. We encourage you to adjust these recipes to suit your own nutritional needs and preferences. Your journey to heart health is personal, and your diet should reflect that.

We highly recommend consulting with your healthcare provider or a registered dietitian before making any significant changes to your diet. They can provide personalized advice and help you navigate any confusion you might encounter along the way. Your doctor knows your health history and can guide you in tailoring these recipes to ensure they are the best fit for you.

Additionally, while we have provided approximate nutritional information for each recipe, please note that these values can vary. Factors such as ingredient brands, portion sizes, and preparation methods can all influence the final nutritional content. We encourage you to use this information as a guide rather than an exact measure, and consider tracking your own intake if you need precise nutritional data.

Furthermore, If our cookbook has brought joy to your kitchen and table, we'd be thrilled to hear about your experiences in an Amazon review. On the flip side, if you stumble upon any hiccups while exploring our recipes, don't hesitate to get in touch at **kloppkingsley@gmail.com.** We're here to support your cooking journey every step of the way

Our goal is to make heart-healthy eating an enjoyable and sustainable part of your life. We hope you find inspiration, comfort, and nourishment in the recipes within this book. Remember, this is a starting point, and you have the freedom to adapt and evolve these meals to better suit your personal journey.

Introduction..

Welcome to a journey of taste, health, and heart! Imagine a world where every meal not only satisfies your hunger but also supports your heart health, particularly if you're living with atrial fibrillation (AFib). This cookbook is your companion, designed specifically for beginners like you who are eager to explore the wonderful world of heart-healthy eating. Whether you're newly diagnosed or looking to improve your diet, "AFib Diet Cookbook for Beginners" is here to transform your kitchen into a haven of wellness and deliciousness. You might be thinking, "Can my diet really impact my AFib?" The answer is a resounding yes! What you eat plays a significant role in managing AFib, a condition characterized by an irregular and often rapid heart rate. The right diet can help reduce symptoms, improve overall heart health, and even prevent further complications. This cookbook is packed with recipes that are not only easy to make but also filled with ingredients that support heart health, ensuring you get the best nutrition possible without sacrificing flavor.

Let's start with a little heart-to-heart about AFib. Living with this condition means you have to be more mindful of your lifestyle choices, and diet is a big part of that. But don't worry, healthy eating doesn't have to be boring or restrictive. This book is all about showing you how to create mouth-watering meals that are good for your heart and easy to prepare. We've taken the guesswork out of meal planning by providing simple, delicious recipes that you'll look forward to making and eating.
Picture this: You wake up to the aroma of a hearty, satisfying breakfast—maybe it's a warm bowl of oatmeal topped with fresh berries and a sprinkle of nuts. For lunch, you could enjoy a vibrant, colorful salad filled with leafy greens, crunchy vegetables, and a zesty lemon dressing. Dinner might be a perfectly grilled piece of fish, seasoned with herbs and spices, accompanied by a side of roasted sweet potatoes and steamed broccoli. Each recipe in this book is designed to be nutritious, easy to make, and absolutely delicious.

One of the best things about the recipes in this cookbook is their simplicity. You don't need to be a gourmet chef to prepare these dishes. We've made sure that the ingredients are easy to find and the steps are straightforward. Even if you're a beginner in the kitchen, you'll find that cooking heart-healthy meals is not only doable but also enjoyable. Each recipe comes with clear instructions and helpful tips to make your cooking experience smooth and fun.

We understand that starting a new diet can be intimidating, especially when dealing with a health condition like AFib. That's why we've included a variety of recipes to suit all tastes and preferences. From hearty breakfasts and light lunches to satisfying dinners and delectable desserts, there's something for everyone. You'll discover that healthy eating can be diverse and exciting, filled with a variety of flavors and textures. Beyond the recipes, this book is packed with valuable information to help you on your heart-health journey. We'll guide you through the basics of AFib, explaining how different foods affect your heart and why certain ingredients are beneficial. You'll learn about the importance of maintaining a balanced diet rich in fruits, vegetables, lean proteins, whole grains, and healthy fats. We also provide tips on meal planning, shopping for heart-healthy ingredients, and making smart choices when dining out.

But it's not just about what you eat; it's about embracing a lifestyle that supports your overall well-being. We encourage you to pair your healthy diet with other heart-friendly habits like regular physical activity, stress management, and staying hydrated. This holistic approach can make a significant difference in managing your AFib and improving your quality of life. As you set out on this culinary adventure, remember that every small change you make is a step towards better heart health. It's about progress, not perfection. With **AFib Diet Cookbook for Beginners,** you have all the tools you need to start creating delicious, heart-healthy meals that you and your loved ones will enjoy. So, tie on your apron, grab your favorite knife, and get ready to cook up some goodness for your heart. Your journey to a healthier, happier heart starts now. Let's get cooking!

Part 1

What is Atrial Fibrillation (AFib)?

Understanding AFib

Atrial Fibrillation, commonly known as AFib, is more than just a medical condition—it's a daily companion that reshapes your life in unexpected ways. Imagine your heart, a robust and tireless worker, suddenly struggling to keep a steady beat. That's AFib. It disrupts the natural rhythm of your heart, transforming the familiar "lub-dub" into a chaotic flutter, like a butterfly trapped in a jar.

But let's step back for a moment and appreciate the marvel that is the human heart. This fist-sized powerhouse tirelessly pumps blood, supplying oxygen and nutrients to every cell in your body. It's a symphony of precision, with each beat harmoniously orchestrated by electrical impulses. AFib throws a wrench into this finely tuned machine, causing the upper chambers of the heart (the atria) to quiver rather than contract properly. When you have AFib, those electrical impulses that usually fire in perfect sync become erratic. It's as if the conductor of an orchestra suddenly lost control, leading to a disjointed and unpredictable performance. This irregularity can cause your heart to race, slow down, or beat unevenly. The physical sensation might feel like your heart is flip-flopping, pounding, or skipping beats—an unnerving experience that can leave you feeling anxious and out of control. Understanding AFib also means recognizing the impact it has beyond the physical symptoms. It's the emotional toll of living with a condition that can strike at any moment, the uncertainty of not knowing when your heart might start racing again. It's the lifestyle adjustments, the medications, and the constant vigilance over what you eat and how you live. It's the conversations with loved ones, explaining why you might need to rest more often or why you're avoiding certain foods.

But amidst the challenges, understanding AFib also opens the door to empowerment. Knowledge becomes your ally, transforming fear into action. You learn about the importance of a heart-healthy diet, the benefits of regular exercise, and the need to manage stress. You discover the value of regular check-ups and the role of medications in keeping your heart's rhythm in check. Living with AFib is a journey of adaptation and resilience. It's about finding balance—literally and figuratively—as you navigate the highs and lows of this condition. And while AFib may be a part of your life, it doesn't define you. With the right tools, support, and mindset, you can manage AFib and continue to live a fulfilling, vibrant life.

So, take heart. Understanding AFib is the first step towards taking control. It's a path to not only managing your health but also rediscovering your strength and capacity for resilience. You're not alone on this journey, and with each beat, you're writing a story of courage and hope.

Symptoms and Risks of AFib

Symptoms of AFib

AFib symptoms can vary widely from person to person, and sometimes, they can be so subtle that they're easily overlooked. However, for many, the symptoms are unmistakable and can significantly impact daily life.

1. Palpitations: One of the most common symptoms is a feeling of your heart racing, fluttering, or pounding. This sensation, known as palpitations, can be sudden and alarming, often described as if your heart is flip-flopping or skipping beats. It can happen during activity or while you're at rest, catching you off guard and leaving you feeling unsettled.
2. Fatigue: AFib can lead to persistent fatigue and a lack of energy. This isn't just ordinary tiredness; it's a deep, overwhelming sense of exhaustion that makes even simple tasks feel monumental. Your body works harder to keep up with the irregular heartbeat, which can drain your energy reserves more quickly.
3. Shortness of Breath: Breathing can become difficult, especially during physical exertion or while lying down. This shortness of breath occurs because your heart's erratic rhythm can impair its ability to pump blood efficiently, leading to a build-up of fluid in the lungs.
4. Dizziness and Fainting: The irregular heartbeat can affect blood flow to your brain, causing dizziness, light-headedness, or even fainting spells. These episodes can be frightening and may restrict your ability to engage in daily activities without fear of suddenly losing consciousness.
5. Chest Pain: Some people with AFib experience chest discomfort or pain. While this can be due to the heart's irregular activity, it's crucial to remember that chest pain can also signal other serious conditions, like a heart attack. Always seek immediate medical attention if you experience chest pain.
6. Anxiety and Panic: The unpredictable nature of AFib can trigger anxiety and panic attacks. The sensation of your heart racing or the fear of an impending episode can be mentally taxing, compounding the physical symptoms with emotional stress.

Risks Associated with AFib

The symptoms of AFib are not just uncomfortable—they can signal underlying risks that need careful management. Understanding these risks can help you take proactive steps to protect your health.

1. Stroke: AFib significantly increases the risk of stroke. The irregular heart rhythm can cause blood to pool in the atria, leading to the formation of blood clots. If a clot travels to the brain, it can block a blood vessel and cause a stroke. This risk makes it essential to manage AFib with medications like blood thinners and regular monitoring.

2. Heart Failure: Chronic AFib can weaken the heart over time, leading to heart failure. The heart's inability to pump blood effectively can result in fluid build-up in the lungs and other parts of the body, causing symptoms like swelling, shortness of breath, and severe fatigue.

3. Cognitive Decline: There's growing evidence that AFib can contribute to cognitive decline and dementia. The irregular blood flow and the risk of small, undetected strokes can impair brain function over time, affecting memory and cognitive abilities.

4. Other Complications: AFib can also lead to other complications, such as chronic fatigue and reduced exercise tolerance. The ongoing struggle to maintain a regular heartbeat can wear down your body, leading to a decreased quality of life and limiting your ability to engage in activities you once enjoyed.

5. Medication Side Effects: Managing AFib often involves medications to control heart rate and prevent blood clots. These medications, while necessary, can have side effects, including increased bleeding risk (from blood thinners), fatigue, and other drug-specific effects. Regular follow-ups with your healthcare provider are crucial to balancing these risks.

Treatment of AFib

Lifestyle Changes

1. Diet and Nutrition: Adopting a heart-healthy diet is foundational in managing AFib. Focus on foods rich in omega-3 fatty acids, such as fish, nuts, and seeds. Incorporate plenty of fruits, vegetables, whole grains, and lean proteins. Reducing salt, sugar, and saturated fats can help control blood pressure and weight, both of which are critical for heart health. Staying hydrated and avoiding excessive alcohol and caffeine can also prevent AFib episodes.
2. Exercise: Regular physical activity strengthens the heart and improves overall cardiovascular health. Aim for a balanced exercise regimen that includes aerobic activities like walking, swimming, or cycling, combined with strength training and flexibility exercises. Always consult your doctor before starting a new exercise program to ensure it's safe for your specific condition.
3. Stress Management: Stress and anxiety can trigger or worsen AFib. Incorporating stress-reducing techniques such as yoga, meditation, deep breathing exercises, and mindfulness can be beneficial. Finding hobbies and activities that bring joy and relaxation is equally important.
4. Avoiding Triggers: Identifying and avoiding triggers that can induce AFib episodes is crucial. Common triggers include excessive caffeine, alcohol, high-stress situations, and certain medications. Keeping a symptom diary can help pinpoint specific triggers and allow you to make necessary adjustments.

Medications

Medications play a vital role in controlling AFib and preventing complications. Your healthcare provider will tailor a medication plan based on your symptoms, overall health, and specific needs.

1. Rate Control Medications: These medications help slow down the heart rate, ensuring it doesn't beat too quickly. Beta-blockers (like metoprolol) and calcium channel blockers (like diltiazem) are commonly prescribed for this purpose.
2. Rhythm Control Medications: These drugs aim to restore and maintain a normal heart rhythm. Antiarrhythmic medications such as amiodarone, flecainide, and sotalol can help manage irregular heartbeats. It's important to monitor for potential side effects, as these medications can sometimes have serious consequences.
3. Anticoagulants (Blood Thinners): To reduce the risk of stroke, blood thinners are often prescribed. Common anticoagulants include warfarin, dabigatran, rivaroxaban, and apixaban. Regular blood tests may be required to monitor the effectiveness and adjust dosages, especially with medications like warfarin.
4. Other Medications: Depending on your overall health, additional medications might be prescribed to manage conditions that can exacerbate AFib, such as hypertension, diabetes, or thyroid disorders.

Medical Procedures

For some, lifestyle changes and medications may not be sufficient to manage AFib effectively. In such cases, various medical procedures can offer more direct intervention.

1. Cardioversion: This procedure can be performed electrically or pharmacologically. Electrical cardioversion involves delivering a controlled electric shock to the heart to reset its rhythm. Pharmacological cardioversion uses medications to achieve the same goal. Cardioversion is typically performed in a hospital setting and is often successful in restoring normal rhythm.

2. Catheter Ablation: In this minimally invasive procedure, catheters are threaded through blood vessels to the heart, where heat (radiofrequency) or cold (cryoablation) is used to destroy small areas of heart tissue that are causing irregular electrical signals. Catheter ablation is often recommended for patients who do not respond to medications or cardioversion.

3. Pacemaker: A pacemaker is a small device implanted under the skin of the chest that helps control abnormal heart rhythms. It sends electrical impulses to prompt the heart to beat at a normal rate. Pacemakers are particularly useful for those with bradycardia (a condition where the heart beats too slowly).

4. Surgical Procedures: In some cases, more invasive surgical procedures like the Maze procedure may be recommended. This involves creating a pattern of scar tissue in the heart to disrupt abnormal electrical pathways. It's often performed during other cardiac surgeries, such as valve repair or coronary artery bypass grafting.

Regular Monitoring and Follow-Up

Regular follow-ups with your healthcare provider are essential to managing AFib effectively. This ongoing care includes:

1. Routine Check-Ups: Regular visits to your cardiologist to monitor your heart's rhythm, review medication effectiveness, and adjust treatment plans as needed.

2. Diagnostic Tests: Periodic ECGs, Holter monitors, and echocardiograms can help track the heart's electrical activity and structural health.

3. Blood Tests: For those on anticoagulants, regular blood tests ensure medication levels remain therapeutic without increasing bleeding risk.

Part 2
The AFib Diet Explained
Importance of Diet in Managing AFib

Diet plays a pivotal role in managing Atrial Fibrillation (AFib), influencing both the frequency of episodes and overall heart health. What you eat can have a profound impact on your cardiovascular system, affecting everything from blood pressure and cholesterol levels to inflammation and weight.

Nutritional Foundations for AFib Management
1. Heart-Healthy Foods: Embracing a heart-healthy diet means prioritizing foods that support cardiovascular function. This includes a variety of fruits, vegetables, whole grains, lean proteins, and healthy fats. These foods provide essential nutrients and antioxidants that help protect the heart and reduce inflammation.
2. Omega-3 Fatty Acids: Omega-3 fatty acids, found in fatty fish like salmon, mackerel, and sardines, as well as in flaxseeds, chia seeds, and walnuts, have been shown to benefit heart health. They help reduce inflammation, lower blood pressure, and improve overall heart rhythm stability, making them crucial in an AFib-friendly diet.
3. Fiber-Rich Foods: High-fiber foods like whole grains, legumes, fruits, and vegetables can help manage cholesterol levels and maintain a healthy weight. Soluble fiber, in particular, helps reduce LDL (bad) cholesterol, which is beneficial for heart health.
4. Potassium-Rich Foods: Potassium helps regulate heart function and blood pressure. Foods rich in potassium, such as bananas, oranges, sweet potatoes, spinach, and avocados, should be included in your diet. However, those with kidney issues or who are on certain medications should consult their doctor regarding potassium intake.

Foods to Avoid or Limit
1. High-Sodium Foods: Excess sodium can lead to high blood pressure, a major risk factor for AFib. Processed foods, canned soups, fast food, and salty snacks often contain high levels of sodium. Opt for fresh, unprocessed foods and use herbs and spices to flavor your meals instead of salt.

2. Sugary Foods and Beverages: High sugar intake can contribute to weight gain and insulin resistance, both of which can increase the risk of AFib. Limiting sweets, sugary drinks, and processed snacks can help maintain a healthy weight and reduce the burden on your heart.

3. Saturated and Trans Fats: These unhealthy fats, found in red meat, full-fat dairy products, fried foods, and many processed snacks, can raise cholesterol levels and promote inflammation. Choose healthy fats from sources like olive oil, avocados, nuts, and seeds instead.

4. Alcohol and Caffeine: Both alcohol and caffeine can trigger AFib episodes in some people. It's wise to limit alcohol intake and be mindful of caffeine consumption. Some individuals may need to avoid these entirely to prevent AFib episodes.

Specific Dietary Approaches

1. Mediterranean Diet: The Mediterranean diet, rich in fruits, vegetables, whole grains, nuts, seeds, and olive oil, has been shown to improve heart health and reduce the risk of AFib. It emphasizes healthy fats, lean proteins, and a variety of plant-based foods, making it an ideal dietary approach for managing AFib.

2. DASH Diet: The Dietary Approaches to Stop Hypertension (DASH) diet focuses on reducing sodium intake and eating nutrient-rich foods that lower blood pressure. This diet includes plenty of fruits, vegetables, whole grains, and lean proteins while limiting sweets, red meats, and fats.

3. Anti-Inflammatory Diet: Chronic inflammation is linked to various heart conditions, including AFib. An anti-inflammatory diet includes foods that fight inflammation, such as leafy greens, berries, fatty fish, nuts, and seeds, while avoiding processed foods, refined sugars, and trans fats.

Hydration

Proper hydration is essential for heart health. Dehydration can lead to electrolyte imbalances, which can trigger AFib episodes. Aim to drink plenty of water throughout the day, and be cautious with beverages that can dehydrate you, such as caffeinated and alcoholic drinks.

Managing Weight

Maintaining a healthy weight is crucial for managing AFib. Excess weight can strain the heart and increase the risk of AFib episodes. A balanced diet combined with regular physical activity can help you achieve and maintain a healthy weight, reducing the frequency and severity of AFib symptoms.

Role of Nutrients and Supplements in Managing AFib

Managing Atrial Fibrillation (AFib) effectively involves not only lifestyle changes and medical treatments but also a keen focus on proper nutrition. Essential nutrients and supplements play a significant role in maintaining heart health, reducing the frequency of AFib episodes, and minimizing the risk of complications.

Essential Nutrients for Heart Health

1. **Omega-3 Fatty Acids**

Omega-3 fatty acids are vital for heart health due to their anti-inflammatory properties and ability to improve heart rhythm. These fatty acids help reduce triglycerides, lower blood pressure, and decrease the risk of abnormal heartbeats.

- Sources: Fatty fish (salmon, mackerel, sardines), flaxseeds, chia seeds, walnuts, and supplements (fish oil capsules).
- Recommended Intake: Aim for at least two servings of fatty fish per week or consider a fish oil supplement if dietary intake is insufficient.

2. Magnesium

Magnesium is crucial for maintaining normal muscle and nerve function, including heart rhythm regulation. It helps prevent irregular heartbeats by stabilizing the electrical activity of the heart.

- Sources: Leafy green vegetables (spinach, kale), nuts and seeds (almonds, pumpkin seeds), whole grains, legumes, and supplements.
- Recommended Intake: The daily recommended amount varies by age and gender, typically around 400-420 mg for men and 310-320 mg for women. Consult your healthcare provider for personalized advice.

3. Potassium

Potassium helps balance electrolytes and maintain proper heart function. It is particularly important for those taking certain medications that can deplete potassium levels.

- Sources: Bananas, oranges, sweet potatoes, spinach, avocados, and supplements.
- Recommended Intake: The recommended daily intake is about 2,500-3,000 mg for adults. High potassium foods should be balanced with any dietary restrictions or medications.

4. Calcium

Calcium is essential for heart muscle contraction and maintaining a steady heartbeat. However, balance is key, as excessive calcium without adequate magnesium can contribute to arrhythmias.

- Sources: Dairy products, leafy greens, fortified plant-based milks, and supplements.
- Recommended Intake: Adults typically need about 1,000-1,200 mg per day, but this should be adjusted based on individual dietary intake and health needs.

5. Fiber

Dietary fiber helps manage cholesterol levels and maintain a healthy weight, both important for heart health. Soluble fiber, in particular, can lower LDL cholesterol.

- Sources: Whole grains, fruits, vegetables, legumes, nuts, and seeds.
- Recommended Intake: Aim for at least 25-30 grams of fiber per day.

Beneficial Supplements for AFib

1. Coenzyme Q10 (CoQ10)

CoQ10 is a powerful antioxidant that supports energy production in cells, including heart muscle cells. It can help improve heart function and reduce the frequency of AFib episodes.

- Sources: Found in small amounts in fatty fish, organ meats, and whole grains; more commonly taken as a supplement.
- Dosage: Typical dosages range from 100 to 200 mg per day. Consult your healthcare provider for appropriate dosing.

2. Vitamin D

Vitamin D is essential for cardiovascular health. Low levels of vitamin D have been associated with an increased risk of cardiovascular diseases, including AFib.

- Sources: Sunlight exposure, fatty fish, fortified dairy products, and supplements.
- Dosage: The recommended daily intake is about 600-800 IU, but higher doses may be needed for those with a deficiency. A blood test can determine your levels and help guide supplementation.

3. B Vitamins

B vitamins, particularly B6, B12, and folate, are important for reducing homocysteine levels, an amino acid linked to heart disease risk.

- Sources: Whole grains, meat, eggs, dairy products, leafy greens, and supplements.
- Dosage: Daily requirements vary, with folate at 400 mcg, B6 at 1.3-2 mg, and B12 at 2.4 mcg for most adults. Supplementation needs can vary based on dietary intake and health status.

4. L-Carnitine

L-Carnitine is an amino acid derivative that helps with energy production in heart cells. It has been shown to improve heart function and may benefit those with AFib.

- Sources: Found in meat and dairy products; also available as a supplement.
- Dosage: Common dosages range from 500 to 2,000 mg per day. Consult your healthcare provider for personalized advice.

Balancing Nutrients and Supplements

While supplements can be beneficial, they should not replace a balanced diet. It's important to focus on whole foods to obtain essential nutrients naturally. Supplements should be considered an adjunct to, not a replacement for, a healthy diet. Additionally, always consult your healthcare provider before starting any new supplements, especially if you are taking medications or have other health conditions.

Interactions and Precautions

1. Medication Interactions: Some supplements can interact with medications used to treat AFib or other conditions. For example, blood thinners like warfarin can interact with vitamin K, which is found in leafy greens and some supplements.
2. Over-Supplementation: Taking too much of certain vitamins and minerals can be harmful. For instance, excessive calcium without adequate magnesium can cause heart rhythm issues.
3. Personalized Advice: Individual needs can vary significantly. A registered dietitian or healthcare provider can help tailor your nutrient and supplement intake based on your specific health needs and lifestyle.

Breakfast Recipes

1. Apple Cinnamon Oatmeal
Ingredients
- 1 cup rolled oats
- 2 cups water
- 1 apple, peeled, cored, and diced
- 1 teaspoon ground cinnamon
- 1 tablespoon honey or maple syrup
- 1/4 cup chopped walnuts
- 1/4 teaspoon vanilla extract

Instructions
1. In a medium saucepan, bring water to a boil.
2. Add oats, diced apple, and cinnamon. Reduce heat to a simmer.
3. Cook for about 5 minutes, stirring occasionally until the oats are tender and the apples are softened.
4. Stir in honey or maple syrup and vanilla extract.
5. Serve hot, topped with chopped walnuts.

Nutrition Info per Serving
- Calories: 320
- Carbohydrates: 54g
- Protein: 6g
- Fat: 10g
- Fiber: 8g
- Sodium: 5mg

Serves
2
Cooking Time
15 minutes

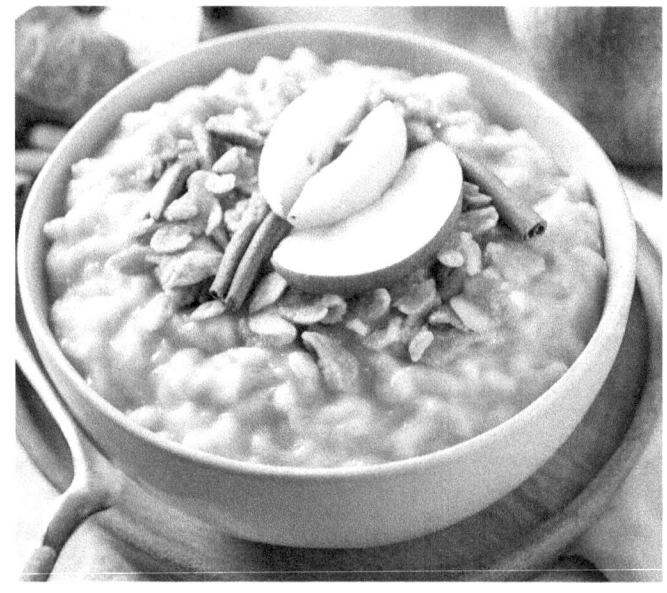

2. Banana Nut Oatmeal

Ingredients

- 1 cup rolled oats
- 2 cups almond milk (unsweetened)
- 1 banana, sliced
- 1/4 cup chopped almonds
- 1 tablespoon chia seeds
- 1 teaspoon ground cinnamon
- 1 tablespoon honey or maple syrup

Instructions

1. In a medium saucepan, bring almond milk to a boil.
2. Add oats and reduce heat to a simmer.
3. Cook for about 5 minutes, stirring occasionally until the oats are tender.
4. Stir in sliced banana, chopped almonds, chia seeds, cinnamon, and honey or maple syrup.
5. Serve hot.

Nutrition Info per Serving

- Calories: 350
- Carbohydrates: 56g
- Protein: 8g
- Fat: 12g
- Fiber: 9g
- Sodium: 95mg

Serves

2

Cooking Time

10 minutes

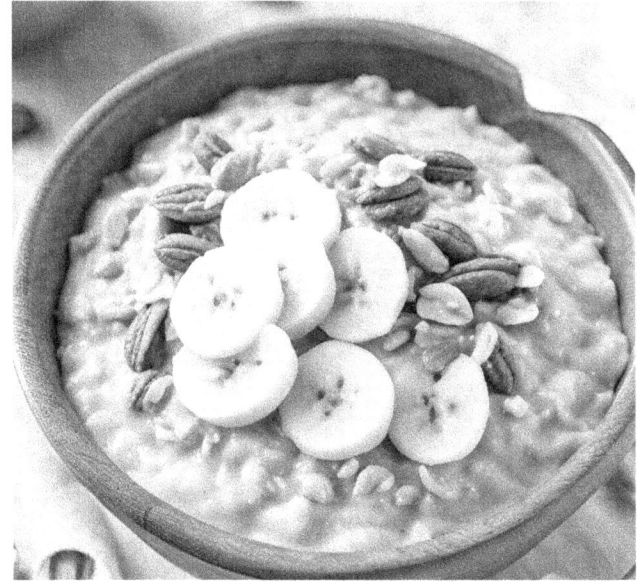

3. Berry Oatmeal Smoothie
Ingredients
- 1/2 cup rolled oats
- 1 cup almond milk (unsweetened)
- 1/2 cup mixed berries (fresh or frozen)
- 1 banana
- 1 tablespoon chia seeds
- 1 tablespoon honey or maple syrup
- 1/2 teaspoon vanilla extract

Instructions
1. In a blender, combine all ingredients.
2. Blend until smooth and creamy.
3. Pour into glasses and serve immediately.

Nutrition Info per Serving
- Calories: 300
- Carbohydrates: 60g
- Protein: 5g
- Fat: 7g
- Fiber: 9g
- Sodium: 85mg

Serves
2
Cooking Time
5 minutes

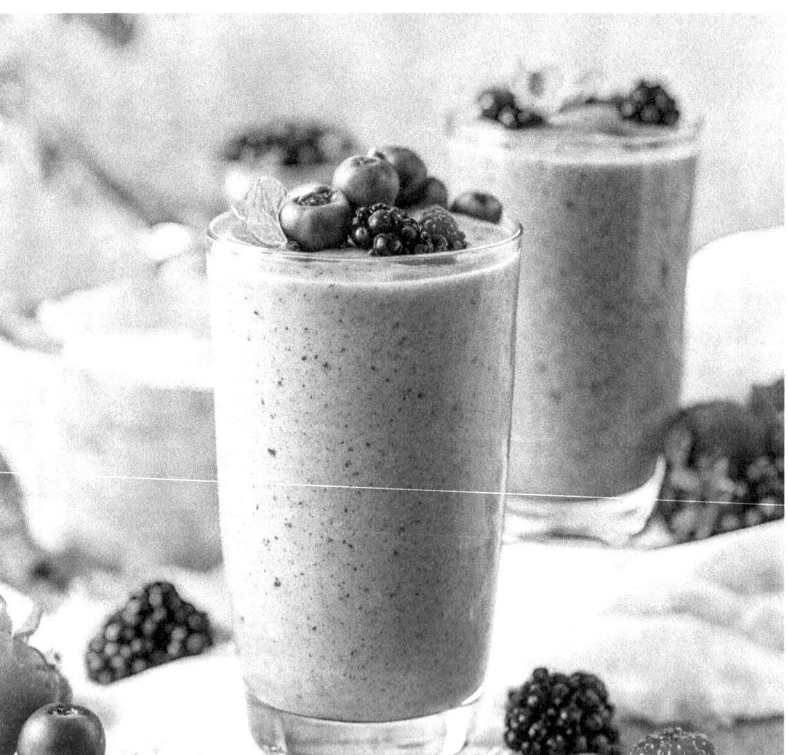

4. Vegetable Frittata
Ingredients
- 6 large eggs
- 1/2 cup milk (dairy or non-dairy)
- 1 cup spinach, chopped
- 1/2 cup cherry tomatoes, halved
- 1/2 cup bell pepper, diced
- 1/4 cup onion, finely chopped
- 1/4 cup feta cheese, crumbled
- 1 teaspoon dried oregano
- 1 tablespoon olive oil

Instructions
1. Preheat the oven to 375°F (190°C).
2. In a large bowl, whisk together eggs and milk.
3. Heat olive oil in an oven-safe skillet over medium heat.
4. Add onion and bell pepper, cooking until softened, about 5 minutes.
5. Stir in spinach and cherry tomatoes, cooking for another 2 minutes.
6. Pour egg mixture over the vegetables. Sprinkle with oregano and feta cheese.
7. Transfer the skillet to the preheated oven and bake for 15-20 minutes, or until the eggs are set and slightly golden.
8. Allow to cool for a few minutes before slicing and serving.

Nutrition Info per Serving
- Calories: 180
- Carbohydrates: 5g
- Protein: 12g
- Fat: 13g
- Fiber: 2g
- Sodium: 210mg

Serves
4
Cooking Time
30 minutes

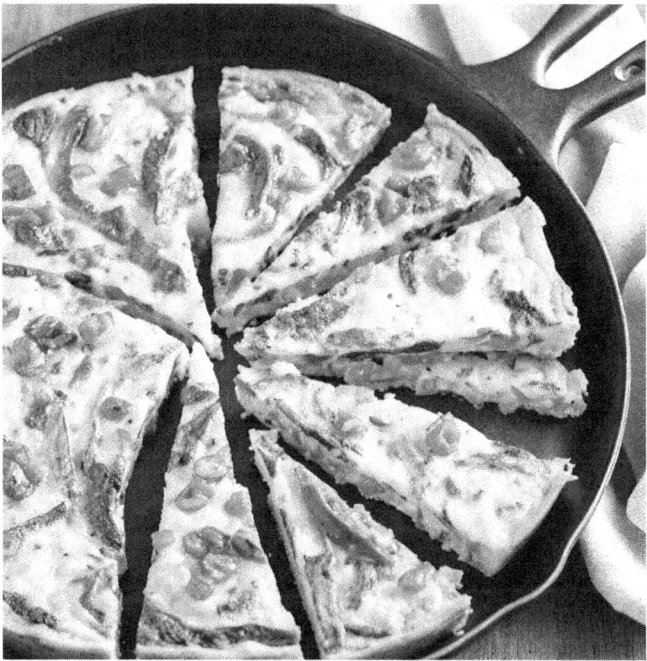

5. Spinach and Mushroom Omelette

Ingredients

- 3 large eggs
- 1/4 cup milk (dairy or non-dairy)
- 1/2 cup spinach, chopped
- 1/2 cup mushrooms, sliced
- 1/4 cup onion, finely chopped
- 1/4 cup shredded mozzarella cheese
- 1 tablespoon olive oil
- 1/2 teaspoon garlic powder

Instructions

1. In a small bowl, whisk together eggs, milk, and garlic powder.
2. Heat olive oil in a non-stick skillet over medium heat.
3. Add onions and mushrooms, cooking until softened, about 5 minutes.
4. Stir in spinach and cook until wilted, about 1-2 minutes.
5. Pour egg mixture over the vegetables in the skillet. Cook until the edges start to set, about 2 minutes.
6. Sprinkle cheese evenly over the omelette.
7. Carefully fold the omelette in half and continue to cook until the eggs are fully set, about 2-3 minutes.
8. Slide the omelette onto a plate and serve hot.

Nutrition Info per Serving

- Calories: 250
- Carbohydrates: 5g
- Protein: 18g
- Fat: 18g
- Fiber: 2g
- Sodium: 250mg

Serves

1

Cooking Time

15 minutes

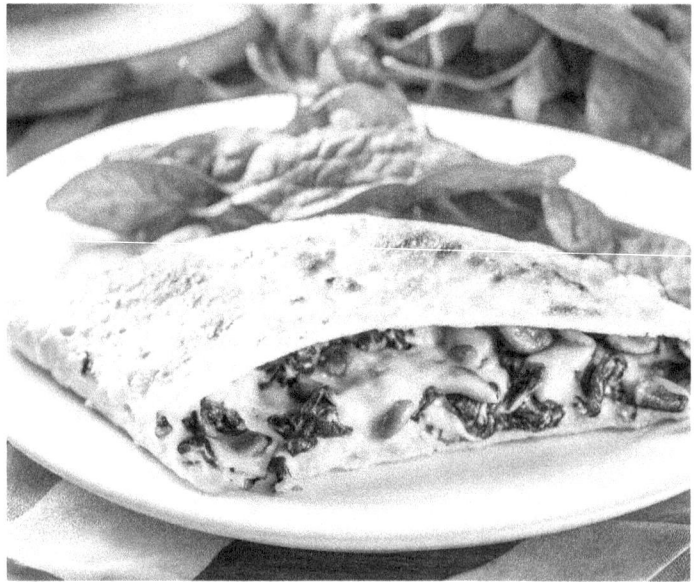

6. Kale and Spinach Smoothie

Ingredients

- 1 cup fresh kale, chopped
- 1 cup fresh spinach
- 1 banana
- 1 cup unsweetened almond milk
- 1 tablespoon chia seeds
- 1 tablespoon honey or maple syrup
- 1/2 teaspoon fresh ginger, grated
- 1/2 cup ice cubes

Instructions

1. In a blender, combine all ingredients.
2. Blend until smooth and creamy.
3. Pour into glasses and serve immediately.

Nutrition Info per Serving

- Calories: 190
- Carbohydrates: 34g
- Protein: 4g
- Fat: 6g
- Fiber: 6g
- Sodium: 80mg

Serves

2

Cooking Time

5 minutes

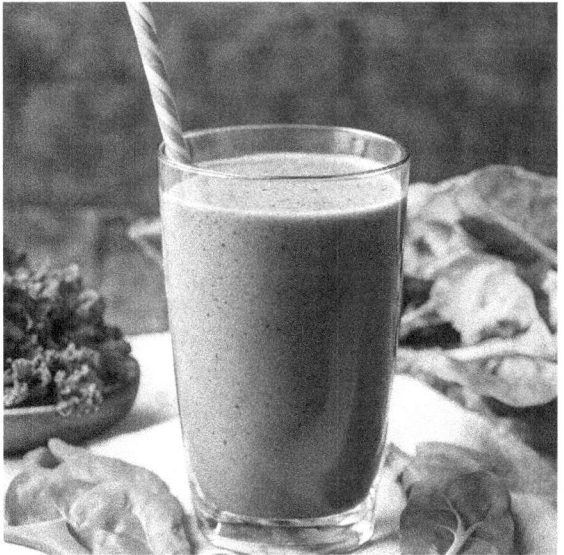

7. Berry Beet Smoothie

Ingredients

- 1 small beet, cooked and peeled
- 1/2 cup mixed berries (strawberries, blueberries, raspberries)
- 1 banana
- 1 cup unsweetened almond milk
- 1 tablespoon chia seeds
- 1 tablespoon honey or maple syrup
- 1/2 cup ice cubes

Instructions

1. In a blender, combine all ingredients.
2. Blend until smooth and creamy.
3. Pour into glasses and serve immediately.

Nutrition Info per Serving

- Calories: 210
- Carbohydrates: 46g
- Protein: 4g
- Fat: 5g
- Fiber: 8g
- Sodium: 100mg

Serves

2

Cooking Time

5 minutes

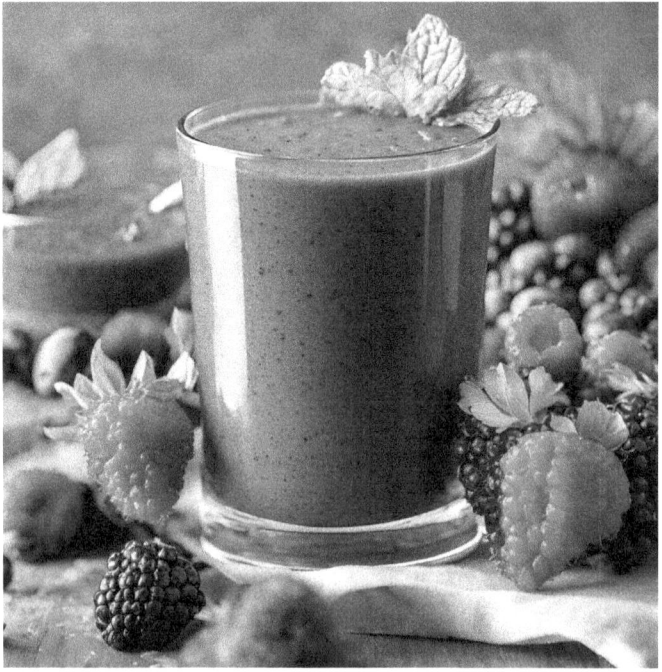

8. Greek Yogurt with Mixed Nuts and Honey
Ingredients
- 2 cups plain Greek yogurt
- 1/4 cup mixed nuts (almonds, walnuts, cashews), chopped
- 2 tablespoons honey
- 1/2 teaspoon ground cinnamon

Instructions
1. Divide the Greek yogurt between two bowls.
2. Top each bowl with chopped mixed nuts.
3. Drizzle each bowl with honey.
4. Sprinkle with ground cinnamon.
5. Serve immediately.

Nutrition Info per Serving
- Calories: 260 Carbohydrates: 23g Protein: 17g Fat: 12g Fiber: 2g
- Sodium: 70mg

Serves
2

Cooking Time
5 minutes

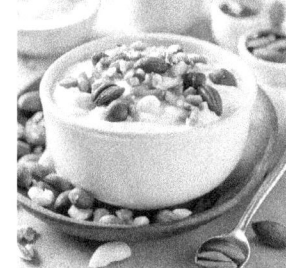

9. Pineapple Turmeric Smoothie
Ingredients
- 1 cup fresh pineapple chunks
- 1 banana
- 1 cup unsweetened coconut milk
- 1/2 teaspoon ground turmeric
- 1 tablespoon chia seeds
- 1 tablespoon honey or maple syrup
- 1/2 cup ice cubes

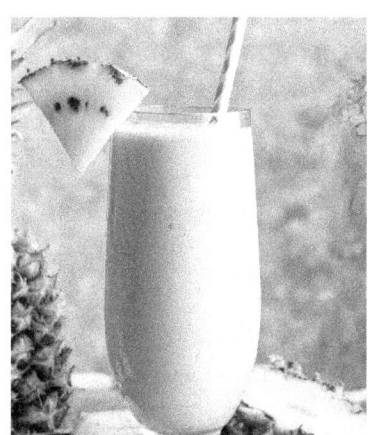

Instructions
1. In a blender, combine all ingredients.
2. Blend until smooth and creamy.
3. Pour into glasses and serve immediately.

Nutrition Info per Serving
- Calories: 200 Carbohydrates: 40g Protein: 3g Fat: 5g Fiber: 6g Sodium: 35mg

Serves
2

Cooking Time
5 minutes

10. Berry Parfait
Ingredients
- 2 cups plain Greek yogurt
- 1 cup mixed berries (strawberries, blueberries, raspberries)
- 1/4 cup granola (low-sugar)
- 2 tablespoons honey
- 1 teaspoon vanilla extract

Instructions
1. In a bowl, mix the Greek yogurt with vanilla extract.
2. In two glasses or bowls, layer the yogurt, berries, and granola.
3. Drizzle each parfait with honey.
4. Serve immediately.

Nutrition Info per Serving
Calories: 290 Carbohydrates: 36g Protein: 16g Fat: 10g Fiber: 4g Sodium: 90mg

Serves
2

Cooking Time
5 minutes

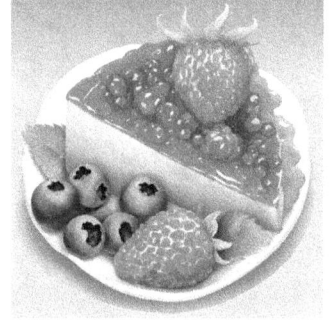

11. Quinoa Breakfast Bowl
Ingredients
- 1 cup quinoa, rinsed
- 2 cups water
- 1/2 cup fresh berries (blueberries, raspberries)
- 1 banana, sliced
- 1/4 cup chopped almonds
- 1 tablespoon chia seeds
- 1 tablespoon honey or maple syrup
- 1/2 teaspoon ground cinnamon

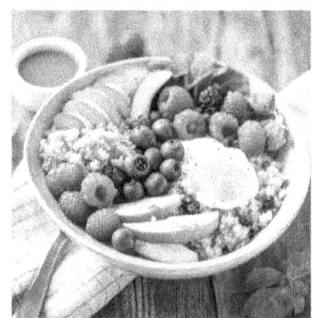

Instructions
1. In a medium saucepan, bring water to a boil.
2. Add quinoa, reduce heat to low, cover, and simmer for 15 minutes or until water is absorbed and quinoa is tender.
3. Divide cooked quinoa into two bowls.
4. Top each bowl with fresh berries, banana slices, chopped almonds, chia seeds, honey or maple syrup, and ground cinnamon.
5. Serve warm.

Nutrition Info per Serving
Calories: 340 Carbohydrates: 58g Protein: 10g   Fat: 10g Fiber: 9g Sodium: 10mg

Serves
2

Cooking Time
20 minutes

12. Whole Wheat Pancakes

Ingredients

- 1 cup whole wheat flour
- 1 tablespoon baking powder
- 1 tablespoon honey
- 1 cup unsweetened almond milk
- 1 large egg
- 1 tablespoon melted coconut oil
- 1 teaspoon vanilla extract

Instructions

1. In a large bowl, whisk together the whole wheat flour and baking powder.
2. In another bowl, whisk together the almond milk, egg, melted coconut oil, honey, and vanilla extract.
3. Pour the wet ingredients into the dry ingredients and stir until just combined.
4. Heat a non-stick skillet over medium heat and lightly grease with a bit of coconut oil.
5. Pour 1/4 cup of batter onto the skillet for each pancake. Cook until bubbles form on the surface, then flip and cook until golden brown on both sides.
6. Serve warm with fresh fruit or a drizzle of maple syrup.

Nutrition Info per Serving

- Calories: 180
- Carbohydrates: 28g
- Protein: 5g
- Fat: 6g
- Fiber: 4g
- Sodium: 270mg

Serves

4 (makes about 8 pancakes)

Cooking Time

20 minutes

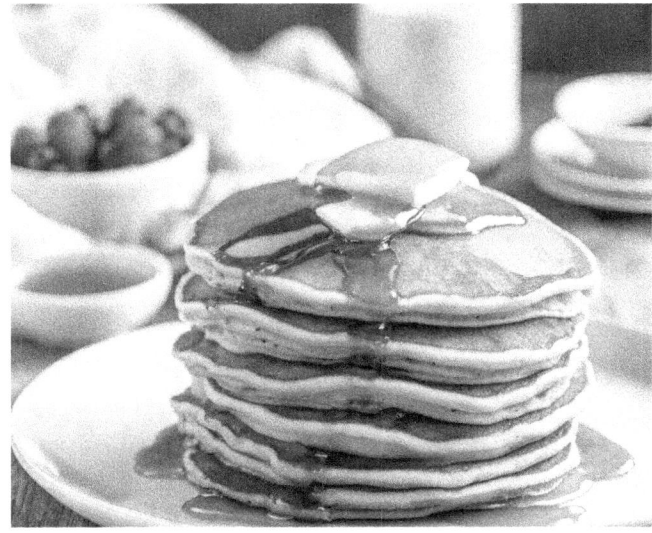

13. Barley Porridge

Ingredients

- 1 cup pearled barley
- 4 cups water
- 1/2 cup almond milk (unsweetened)
- 1 tablespoon honey or maple syrup
- 1 teaspoon ground cinnamon
- 1/4 cup raisins or dried cranberries
- 1/4 cup chopped walnuts

Instructions

1. In a large saucepan, bring water to a boil.
2. Add the barley, reduce heat to low, cover, and simmer for 45 minutes or until barley is tender and most of the water is absorbed.
3. Stir in almond milk, honey or maple syrup, ground cinnamon, raisins or dried cranberries, and chopped walnuts.
4. Serve warm.

Nutrition Info per Serving

- Calories: 220
- Carbohydrates: 45g
- Protein: 5g
- Fat: 4g
- Fiber: 7g
- Sodium: 5mg

Serves
4
Cooking Time
50 minutes

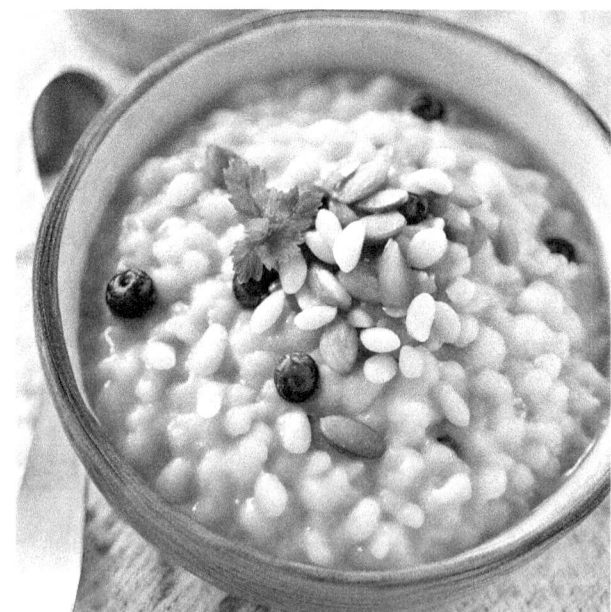

14. Whole Grain Waffles

Ingredients

- 1 1/2 cups whole wheat flour
- 2 teaspoons baking powder
- 1 tablespoon honey
- 1 1/2 cups unsweetened almond milk
- 2 large eggs
- 2 tablespoons melted coconut oil
- 1 teaspoon vanilla extract

Instructions

1. Preheat your waffle iron according to the manufacturer's instructions.
2. In a large bowl, whisk together the whole wheat flour and baking powder.
3. In another bowl, whisk together the almond milk, eggs, melted coconut oil, honey, and vanilla extract.
4. Pour the wet ingredients into the dry ingredients and stir until just combined.
5. Pour the batter into the preheated waffle iron and cook according to the manufacturer's instructions until golden brown and crisp.
6. Serve warm with fresh fruit or a drizzle of maple syrup.

Nutrition Info per Serving

- Calories: 220
- Carbohydrates: 30g
- Protein: 6g
- Fat: 8g
- Fiber: 4g
- Sodium: 240mg

Serves
4 (makes about 8 waffles)
Cooking Time
25 minutes

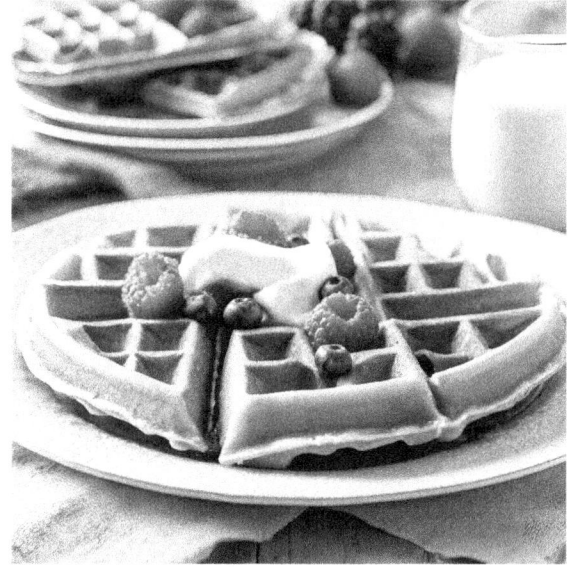

15. Turkey and Spinach Breakfast Sausages

Ingredients

- 1 pound ground turkey
- 1 cup fresh spinach, finely chopped
- 2 garlic cloves, minced
- 1 teaspoon dried oregano
- 1 teaspoon dried thyme
- 1/2 teaspoon smoked paprika
- 1/2 teaspoon ground black pepper
- 1 tablespoon olive oil

Instructions

1. In a large bowl, combine ground turkey, chopped spinach, minced garlic, oregano, thyme, smoked paprika, and black pepper. Mix until well combined.
2. Form the mixture into small patties.
3. Heat olive oil in a large skillet over medium heat.
4. Cook the patties for about 4-5 minutes on each side, or until fully cooked through and golden brown.
5. Serve hot.

Nutrition Info per Serving

- Calories: 180
- Carbohydrates: 2g
- Protein: 23g
- Fat: 9g
- Fiber: 1g
- Sodium: 75mg

Serves
4 (makes about 12 sausages)
Cooking Time
20 minutes

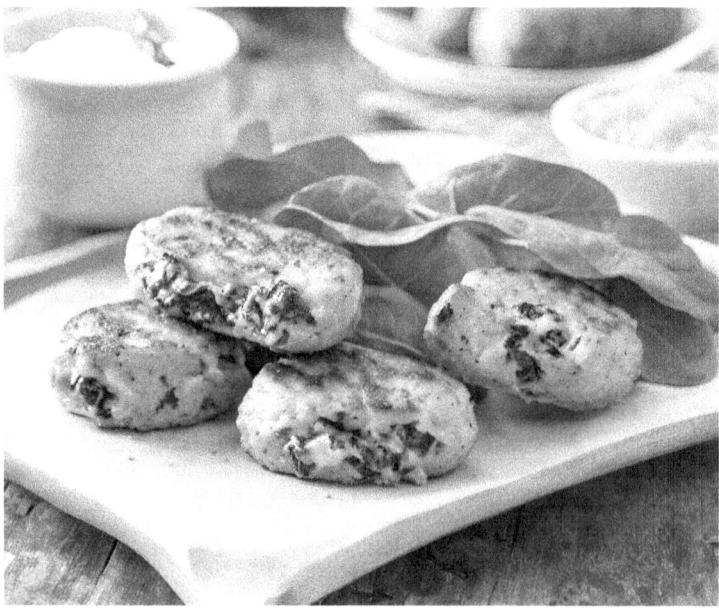

16. Rice Porridge with Berries

Ingredients

- 1 cup brown rice
- 4 cups water
- 1 cup almond milk (unsweetened)
- 1 cup mixed berries (blueberries, strawberries, raspberries)
- 1 tablespoon honey or maple syrup
- 1 teaspoon ground cinnamon
- 1/4 cup sliced almonds

Instructions

1. In a large saucepan, combine brown rice and water. Bring to a boil.
2. Reduce heat to low, cover, and simmer for 40-45 minutes or until rice is tender and water is absorbed.
3. Stir in almond milk, honey or maple syrup, and ground cinnamon. Cook for an additional 5 minutes.
4. Serve warm, topped with mixed berries and sliced almonds.

Nutrition Info per Serving

- Calories: 300
- Carbohydrates: 55g
- Protein: 7g
- Fat: 7g
- Fiber: 6g
- Sodium: 20mg

Serves

4

Cooking Time

50 minutes

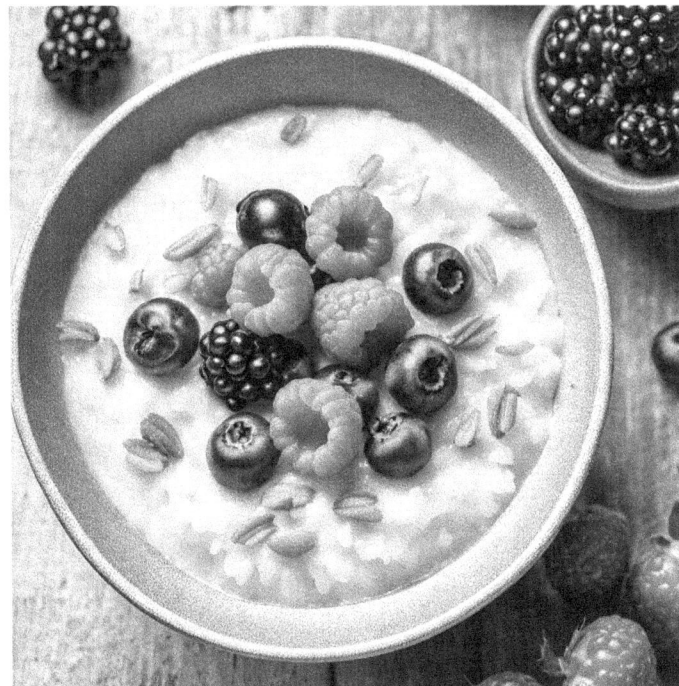

17. Sweet Potato Congee

Ingredients

- 1 cup jasmine rice
- 8 cups water
- 2 medium sweet potatoes, peeled and diced
- 1 tablespoon grated ginger
- 1 tablespoon soy sauce (low sodium)
- 1 tablespoon olive oil
- 1/4 cup chopped green onions

Instructions

1. In a large pot, combine jasmine rice and water. Bring to a boil.
2. Add diced sweet potatoes and grated ginger. Reduce heat to low and simmer for 45-50 minutes, stirring occasionally, until the rice breaks down and the congee thickens.
3. Stir in soy sauce and olive oil.
4. Serve hot, garnished with chopped green onions.

Nutrition Info per Serving

- Calories: 230
- Carbohydrates: 50g
- Protein: 4g
- Fat: 3g
- Fiber: 4g
- Sodium: 200mg

Serves

6

Cooking Time

55 minutes

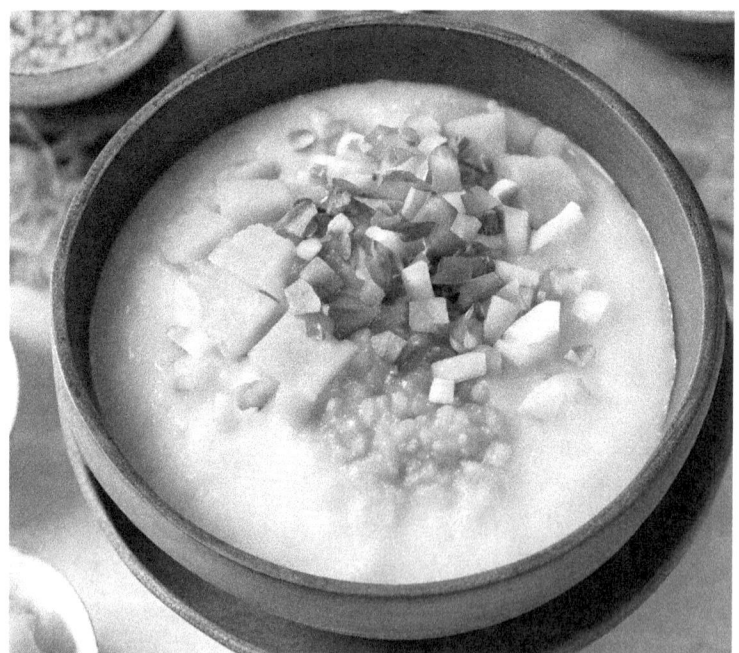

18. Millet Porridge with Apples and Cinnamon

Ingredients

- 1 cup millet
- 3 cups water
- 1 apple, peeled and diced
- 1 cup almond milk (unsweetened)
- 1 tablespoon honey or maple syrup
- 1 teaspoon ground cinnamon
- 1/4 cup chopped walnuts

Instructions

1. In a medium saucepan, combine millet and water. Bring to a boil.
2. Reduce heat to low, cover, and simmer for 20 minutes.
3. Add diced apple, almond milk, honey or maple syrup, and ground cinnamon. Cook for an additional 10 minutes, stirring occasionally, until the millet is tender and the porridge is creamy.
4. Serve warm, topped with chopped walnuts.

Nutrition Info per Serving

- Calories: 270
- Carbohydrates: 45g
- Protein: 6g
- Fat: 8g
- Fiber: 5g
- Sodium: 10mg

Serves

4

Cooking Time

30 minutes

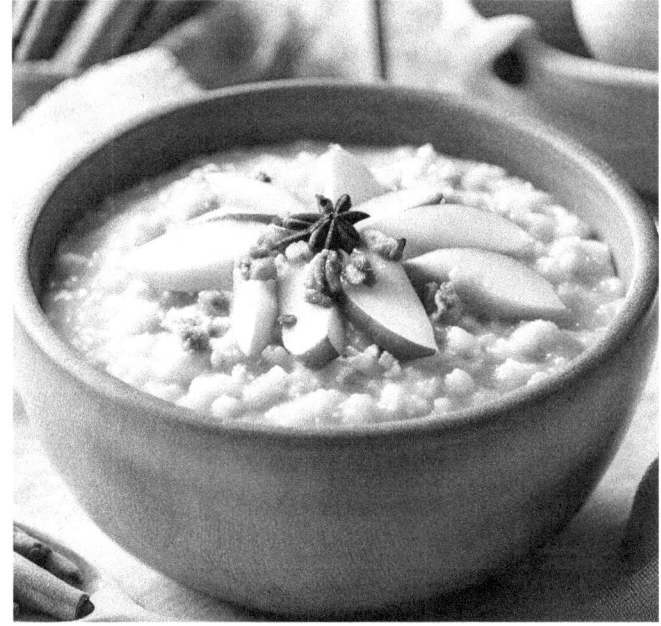

19. Buckwheat Porridge with Honey and Walnuts

Ingredients

- 1 cup buckwheat groats
- 3 cups water
- 1 cup almond milk (unsweetened)
- 1 tablespoon honey
- 1 teaspoon ground cinnamon
- 1/4 cup chopped walnuts

Instructions

1. In a medium saucepan, combine buckwheat groats and water. Bring to a boil.
2. Reduce heat to low, cover, and simmer for 20 minutes, or until buckwheat is tender and water is absorbed.
3. Stir in almond milk, honey, and ground cinnamon. Cook for an additional 5 minutes.
4. Serve warm, topped with chopped walnuts.

Nutrition Info per Serving

- Calories: 260
- Carbohydrates: 43g
- Protein: 7g
- Fat: 8g
- Fiber: 5g
- Sodium: 5mg

Serves

4

Cooking Time

25 minutes

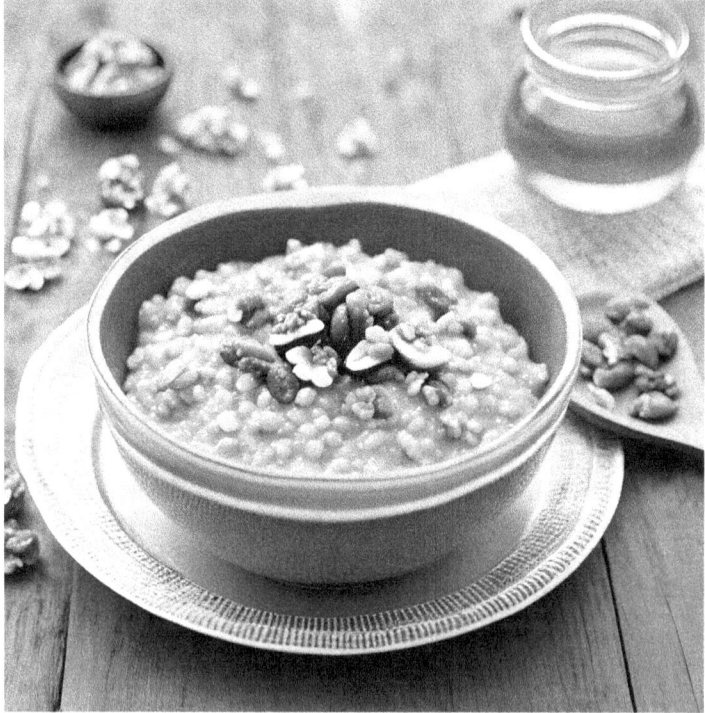

20. Caprese Salad with an Egg

Ingredients

- 2 large tomatoes, sliced
- 1 cup fresh mozzarella, sliced
- 1/2 cup fresh basil leaves
- 4 large eggs
- 2 tablespoons balsamic glaze
- 1 tablespoon olive oil

Instructions

1. Arrange the tomato slices, mozzarella slices, and basil leaves on a plate in alternating layers.
2. Drizzle with olive oil and balsamic glaze.
3. In a medium skillet, cook the eggs sunny-side up or as desired.
4. Place one egg on top of each serving of the salad.
5. Serve immediately.

Nutrition Info per Serving

- Calories: 250
- Carbohydrates: 6g
- Protein: 16g
- Fat: 18g
- Fiber: 2g
- Sodium: 200mg

Serves

4

Cooking Time

15 minutes

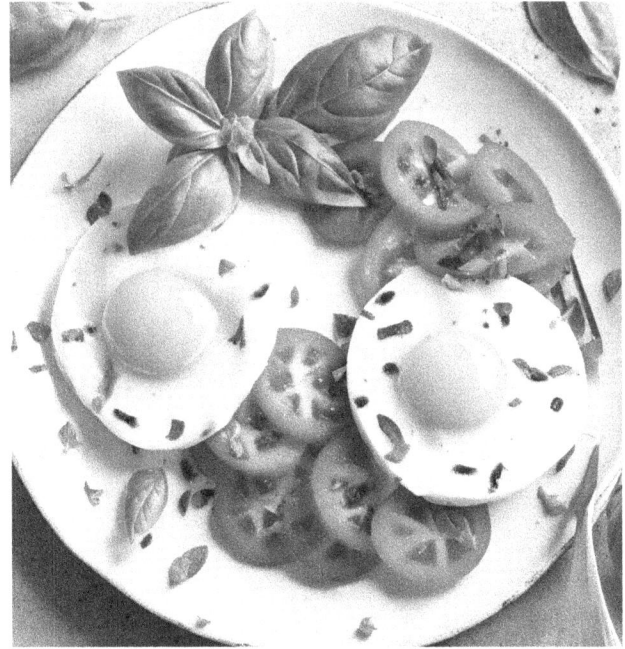

21. Watermelon Salad with Mint and Feta

Ingredients

- 4 cups watermelon, cubed
- 1/2 cup crumbled feta cheese
- 1/4 cup fresh mint leaves, chopped
- 2 tablespoons lime juice
- 1 tablespoon olive oil

Instructions

1. In a large bowl, combine the watermelon cubes and chopped mint leaves.
2. Drizzle with lime juice and olive oil. Toss gently to combine.
3. Sprinkle crumbled feta cheese on top.
4. Serve immediately.

Nutrition Info per Serving

- Calories: 120
- Carbohydrates: 12g
- Protein: 3g
- Fat: 7g
- Fiber: 1g
- Sodium: 150mg

Serves

4

Cooking Time

10 minutes

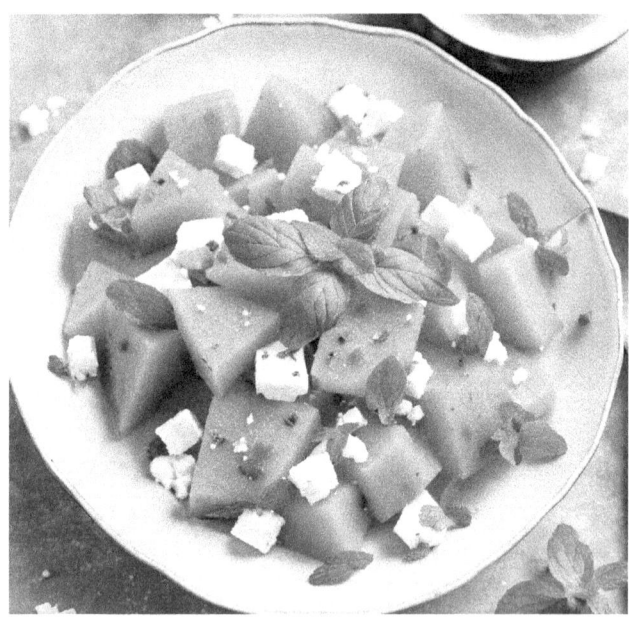

22. Nutty Granola
Ingredients
- 3 cups rolled oats
- 1 cup mixed nuts (almonds, walnuts, pecans), chopped
- 1/2 cup shredded coconut (unsweetened)
- 1/4 cup chia seeds
- 1/4 cup flax seeds
- 1/3 cup honey or maple syrup
- 1/4 cup coconut oil, melted
- 1 teaspoon ground cinnamon
- 1 teaspoon vanilla extract

Instructions
1. Preheat oven to 325°F (165°C).
2. In a large bowl, combine rolled oats, mixed nuts, shredded coconut, chia seeds, and flax seeds.
3. In a small bowl, whisk together honey or maple syrup, melted coconut oil, ground cinnamon, and vanilla extract.
4. Pour the wet mixture over the dry ingredients and stir until well combined.
5. Spread the mixture evenly on a baking sheet lined with parchment paper.
6. Bake for 20-25 minutes, stirring halfway through, until golden brown.
7. Allow to cool completely before storing in an airtight container.

Nutrition Info per Serving
- Calories: 220
- Carbohydrates: 28g
- Protein: 6g
- Fat: 10g
- Fiber: 5g
- Sodium: 10mg

Serves
10
Cooking Time
30 minutes

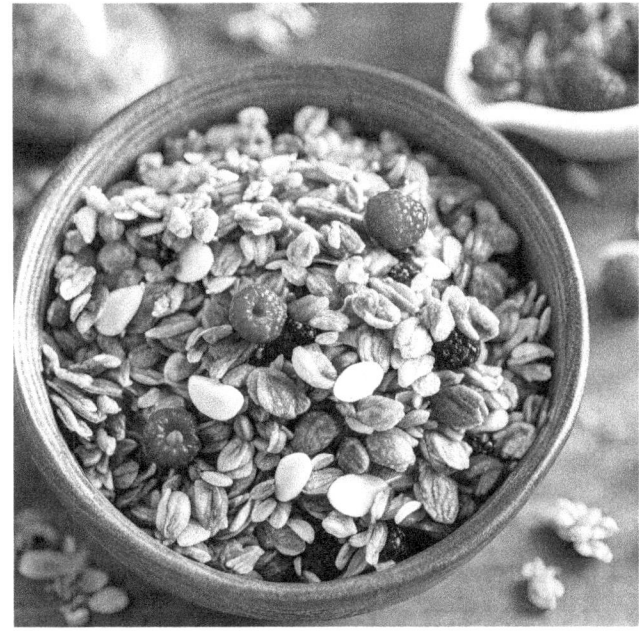

23. Seed Mix Topped Yogurt

Ingredients

- 2 cups plain Greek yogurt
- 1/4 cup pumpkin seeds
- 1/4 cup sunflower seeds
- 2 tablespoons flax seeds
- 2 tablespoons chia seeds
- 1 tablespoon honey or maple syrup
- 1 teaspoon ground cinnamon

Instructions

1. Divide the Greek yogurt into two bowls.
2. In a small bowl, mix together pumpkin seeds, sunflower seeds, flax seeds, and chia seeds.
3. Top each bowl of yogurt with the seed mix.
4. Drizzle with honey or maple syrup and sprinkle with ground cinnamon.
5. Serve immediately.

Nutrition Info per Serving

- Calories: 270
- Carbohydrates: 21g
- Protein: 17g
- Fat: 12g
- Fiber: 5g
- Sodium: 60mg

Serves

2

Cooking Time

5 minutes

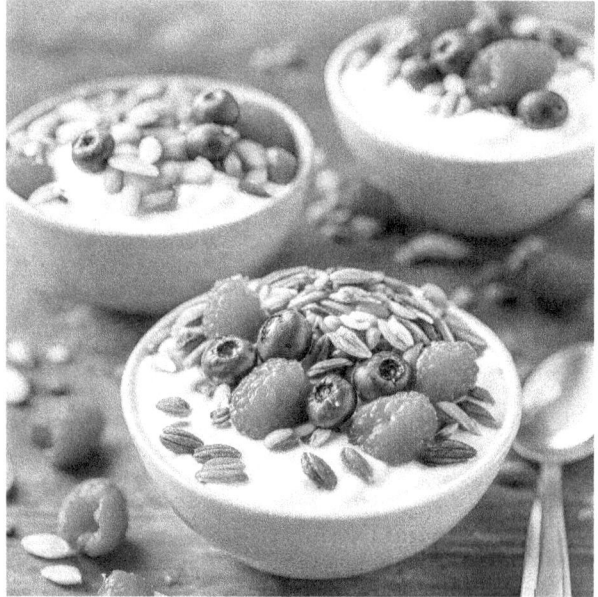

24. Coconut and Almond Chia Breakfast Bowl

Ingredients

- 1/4 cup chia seeds
- 1 cup unsweetened coconut milk
- 1 tablespoon honey or maple syrup
- 1/2 teaspoon vanilla extract
- 1/4 cup sliced almonds
- 1/4 cup unsweetened shredded coconut
- 1/2 cup fresh berries (blueberries, strawberries)

Instructions

1. In a medium bowl, whisk together chia seeds, coconut milk, honey or maple syrup, and vanilla extract.
2. Cover and refrigerate for at least 2 hours or overnight, until the mixture thickens.
3. Divide the chia pudding into two bowls.
4. Top each bowl with sliced almonds, shredded coconut, and fresh berries.
5. Serve chilled.

Nutrition Info per Serving

- Calories: 320
- Carbohydrates: 24g
- Protein: 8g
- Fat: 23g
- Fiber: 12g
- Sodium: 30mg

Serves

2

Cooking Time

5 minutes (plus 2 hours chilling time)

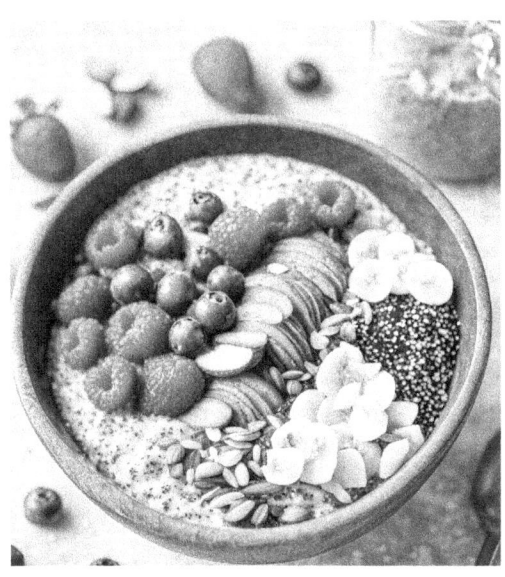

Poultry Recipes

1. Grilled Lemon Herb Chicken

Ingredients

- 4 boneless, skinless chicken breasts
- 1/4 cup olive oil
- 1/4 cup fresh lemon juice
- 3 garlic cloves, minced
- 1 tablespoon fresh thyme leaves
- 1 tablespoon fresh rosemary leaves, chopped
- 1 teaspoon ground black pepper

Instructions

1. In a small bowl, whisk together olive oil, lemon juice, minced garlic, thyme, rosemary, and black pepper.
2. Place the chicken breasts in a large resealable plastic bag or shallow dish.
3. Pour the marinade over the chicken, ensuring each piece is well coated. Marinate in the refrigerator for at least 30 minutes, up to 4 hours.
4. Preheat the grill to medium-high heat.
5. Remove the chicken from the marinade and discard the marinade.
6. Grill the chicken for 6-7 minutes on each side, or until fully cooked and the internal temperature reaches 165°F (75°C).
7. Serve hot.

Nutrition Info per Serving

- Calories: 250
- Carbohydrates: 2g
- Protein: 26g
- Fat: 14g
- Fiber: 0g
- Sodium: 70mg

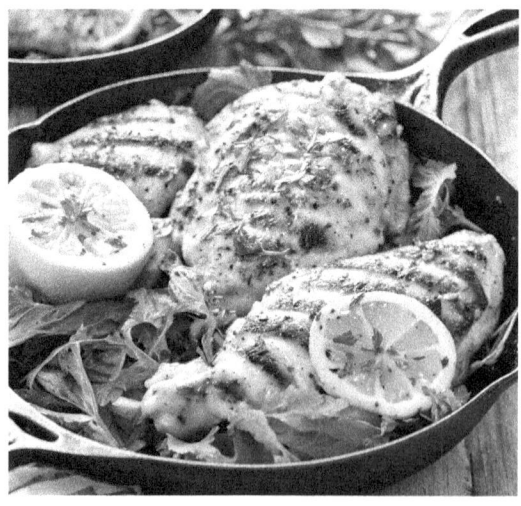

Serves

4

Cooking Time

20 minutes (plus marinating time)

2. Chicken and Vegetable Stir-Fry

Ingredients

- 2 boneless, skinless chicken breasts, sliced thinly
- 2 tablespoons olive oil
- 1 red bell pepper, sliced
- 1 yellow bell pepper, sliced
- 1 cup broccoli florets
- 1 carrot, julienned
- 1 cup snap peas
- 3 garlic cloves, minced
- 1 tablespoon grated ginger
- 1/4 cup low-sodium soy sauce
- 1 tablespoon rice vinegar
- 1 tablespoon honey
- 1 teaspoon sesame oil
- 1 tablespoon sesame seeds (optional)

Instructions

1. In a small bowl, whisk together soy sauce, rice vinegar, honey, and sesame oil. Set aside.
2. Heat olive oil in a large skillet or wok over medium-high heat.
3. Add sliced chicken and cook until no longer pink, about 5-6 minutes.
4. Add minced garlic and grated ginger to the skillet and sauté for 1 minute.
5. Add the bell peppers, broccoli, carrot, and snap peas to the skillet. Stir-fry for about 5-7 minutes, until vegetables are tender-crisp.
6. Pour the soy sauce mixture over the chicken and vegetables, stirring to combine. Cook for an additional 2 minutes.
7. Serve hot, garnished with sesame seeds if desired.

Nutrition Info per Serving

- Calories: 280
- Carbohydrates: 16g
- Protein: 28g
- Fat: 12g
- Fiber: 4g
- Sodium: 450mg

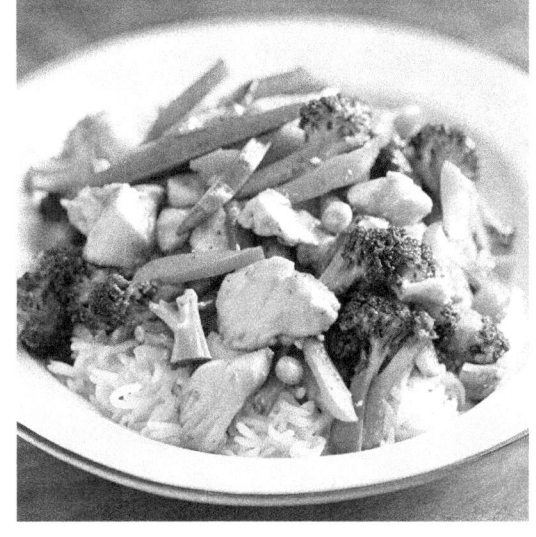

Serves

4

Cooking Time

20 minutes

3. Baked Chicken with Spinach

Ingredients

- 4 boneless, skinless chicken breasts
- 1 tablespoon olive oil
- 3 garlic cloves, minced
- 1 cup fresh spinach, chopped
- 1/2 cup cherry tomatoes, halved
- 1/4 cup feta cheese, crumbled
- 1 teaspoon dried oregano
- 1 teaspoon ground black pepper

Instructions

1. Preheat oven to 375°F (190°C)
2. Heat oliv
3. Add minc
4. Add cho   inutes until spinach i
5. Remove f   o.
6. Season c
7. Place the
8. Transfer   ites, or until the chic   eaches 165°F (75°C).
9. Serve ho

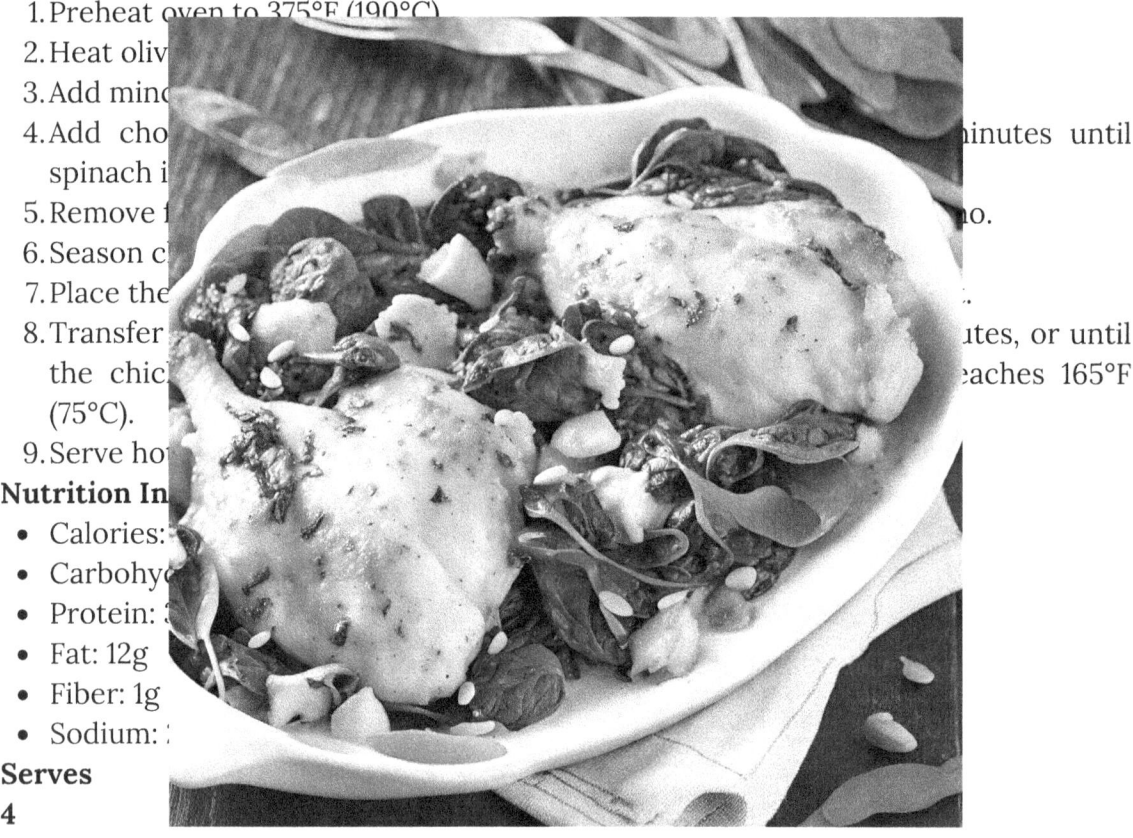

Nutrition In

- Calories:
- Carbohy
- Protein:
- Fat: 12g
- Fiber: 1g
- Sodium:

Serves

4

Cooking Time

40 minutes

4. Chicken Soup with Barley

Ingredients

- 2 boneless, skinless chicken breasts, cubed
- 1 tablespoon olive oil
- 1 onion, chopped
- 3 garlic cloves, minced
- 2 carrots, sliced
- 2 celery stalks, sliced
- 1/2 cup pearl barley
- 6 cups low-sodium chicken broth
- 1 teaspoon dried thyme
- 1 teaspoon dried basil
- 1 bay leaf
- 1 cup spinach, chopped
- 1 teaspoon ground black pepper

Instructions

1. Heat olive oil in a large pot over medium heat.
2. Add chopped onion and sauté for 3-4 minutes until translucent.
3. Add minced garlic, sliced carrots, and sliced celery, cooking for another 5 minutes.
4. Stir in cubed chicken breasts and cook until no longer pink, about 5 minutes.
5. Add pearl barley, chicken broth, dried thyme, dried basil, bay leaf, and ground black pepper to the pot.
6. Bring to a boil, then reduce heat to low and simmer for 30-40 minutes until barley is tender.
7. Stir in chopped spinach and cook for another 5 minutes.
8. Remove the bay leaf before serving.
9. Serve hot.

Nutrition Info per Serving

- Calories: 220
- Carbohydrates: 22g
- Protein: 22g
- Fat: 6g
- Fiber: 5g
- Sodium: 190mg

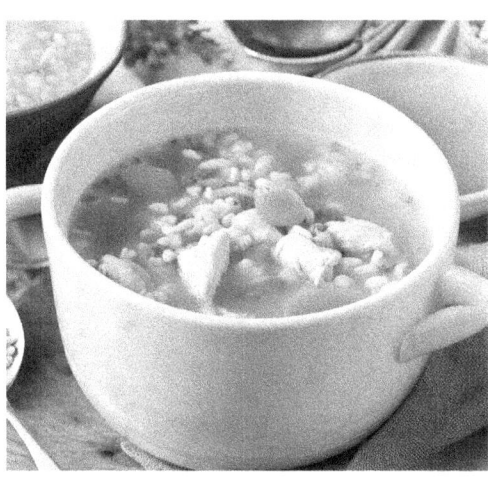

Serves

6

Cooking Time

60 minutes

5. Mediterranean Chicken Salad

Ingredients

- 2 boneless, skinless chicken breasts
- 1 tablespoon olive oil
- 1 teaspoon dried oregano
- 1 teaspoon ground black pepper
- 4 cups mixed greens (spinach, arugula, lettuce)
- 1/2 cup cherry tomatoes, halved
- 1/4 cup Kalamata olives, pitted and sliced
- 1/4 cup cucumber, sliced
- 1/4 cup red onion, thinly sliced
- 1/4 cup feta cheese, crumbled
- 2 tablespoons lemon juice
- 1 tablespoon red wine vinegar

Instructions

1. Preheat grill to medium-high heat.
2. Rub chicken breasts with olive oil, oregano, and ground black pepper.
3. Grill chicken for 6-7 minutes on each side, or until fully cooked and internal temperature reaches 165°F (75°C). Let rest for 5 minutes, then slice thinly.
4. In a large bowl, combine mixed greens, cherry tomatoes, olives, cucumber, red onion, and feta cheese.
5. In a small bowl, whisk together lemon juice and red wine vinegar.
6. Toss the salad with the dressing and top with sliced grilled chicken.
7. Serve immediately.

Nutrition Info per Serving

- Calories: 320
- Carbohydrates: 10g
- Protein: 28g
- Fat: 20g
- Fiber: 3g
- Sodium: 400mg

Serves

4

Cooking Time

20 minutes

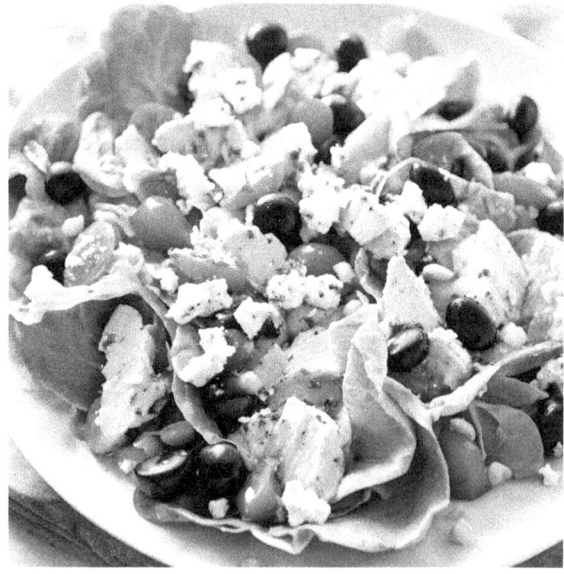

6. Chicken Cacciatore

Ingredients

- 4 boneless, skinless chicken thighs
- 1 tablespoon olive oil
- 1 onion, chopped
- 3 garlic cloves, minced
- 1 bell pepper, sliced
- 1 cup mushrooms, sliced
- 1 can (14.5 ounces) diced tomatoes
- 1/2 cup low-sodium chicken broth
- 1 teaspoon dried oregano
- 1 teaspoon dried basil
- 1/2 teaspoon ground black pepper
- 1/4 cup chopped fresh parsley

Instructions

1. Heat olive oil in a large skillet over medium heat.
2. Add chicken thighs and cook until browned, about 5 minutes on each side. Remove from skillet and set aside.
3. In the same skillet, add chopped onion, minced garlic, bell pepper, and mushrooms. Sauté until vegetables are tender, about 5-7 minutes.
4. Stir in diced tomatoes, chicken broth, oregano, basil, and ground black pepper. Bring to a simmer.
5. Return chicken thighs to the skillet. Cover and simmer for 30 minutes, or until chicken is cooked through and tender.
6. Sprinkle with chopped fresh parsley before serving.
7. Serve hot.

Nutrition Info per Serving

- Calories: 250
- Carbohydrates: 12g
- Protein: 24g
- Fat: 12g
- Fiber: 3g
- Sodium: 300mg

Serves

4

Cooking Time

45 minutes

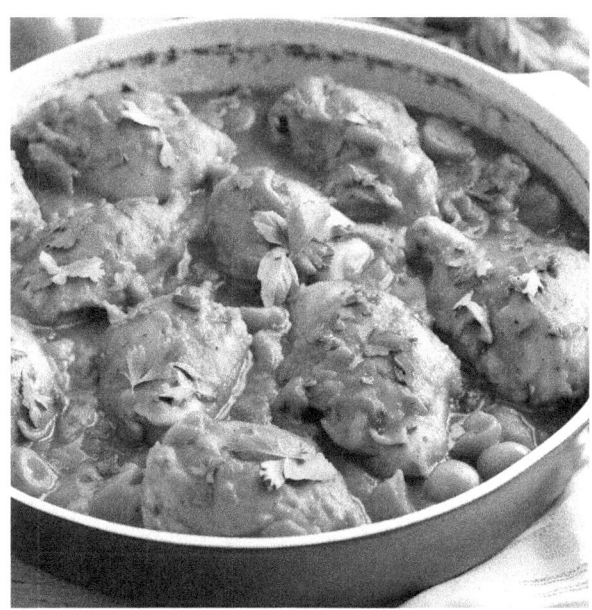

7. Stuffed Chicken Breast

Ingredients

- 4 boneless, skinless chicken breasts
- 1 cup fresh spinach, chopped
- 1/2 cup ricotta cheese
- 1/4 cup sun-dried tomatoes, chopped
- 1 teaspoon dried basil
- 1 teaspoon ground black pepper
- 1 tablespoon olive oil

Instructions

1. Preheat oven to 375°F (190°C).
2. In a medium bowl, mix together chopped spinach, ricotta cheese, sun-dried tomatoes, dried basil, and ground black pepper.
3. Cut a pocket into each chicken breast by slicing horizontally without cutting all the way through.
4. Stuff each chicken breast with the spinach mixture and secure with toothpicks.
5. Heat olive oil in an oven-safe skillet over medium-high heat. Sear each chicken breast for 3-4 minutes on each side until browned.
6. Transfer the skillet to the preheated oven and bake for 20-25 minutes, or until the chicken is cooked through and the internal temperature reaches 165°F (75°C).
7. Remove toothpicks before serving.
8. Serve hot.

Nutrition Info per Serving

- Calories: 300
- Carbohydrates: 5g
- Protein: 36g
- Fat: 15g
- Fiber: 1g
- Sodium: 250mg

Serves

4

Cooking Time

35 minutes

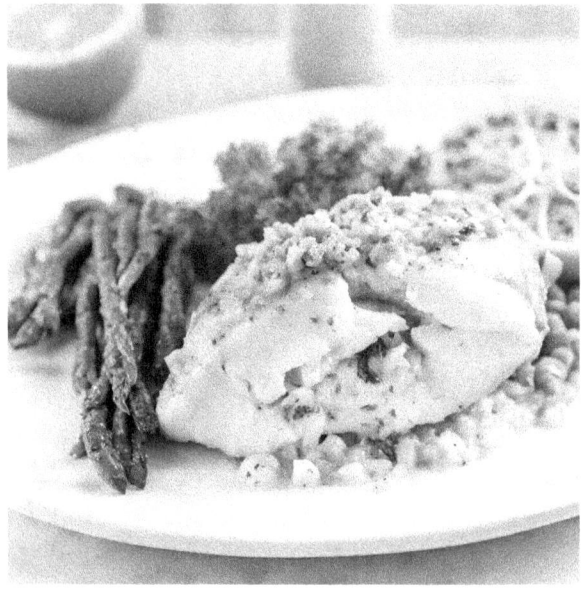

8. Turkey Meatloaf

Ingredients

- 1 pound ground turkey
- 1/2 cup oats
- 1/2 cup onion, finely chopped
- 1/2 cup carrot, grated
- 1/4 cup celery, finely chopped
- 1/4 cup parsley, chopped
- 2 garlic cloves, minced
- 1 egg, beaten
- 1/4 cup ketchup (low sodium)
- 1 teaspoon dried thyme
- 1 teaspoon ground black pepper

Instructions

1. Preheat oven to 350°F (175°C).
2. In a large bowl, combine ground turkey, oats, onion, carrot, celery, parsley, minced garlic, beaten egg, ketchup, dried thyme, and ground black pepper. Mix until well combined.
3. Transfer the mixture to a loaf pan and shape into a loaf.
4. Bake for 45-50 minutes, or until the internal temperature reaches 165°F (75°C).
5. Let the meatloaf rest for 5 minutes before slicing.
6. Serve hot.

Nutrition Info per Serving

- Calories: 220
- Carbohydrates: 12g
- Protein: 26g
- Fat: 8g
- Fiber: 2g
- Sodium: 300mg

Serves

6

Cooking Time

55 minutes

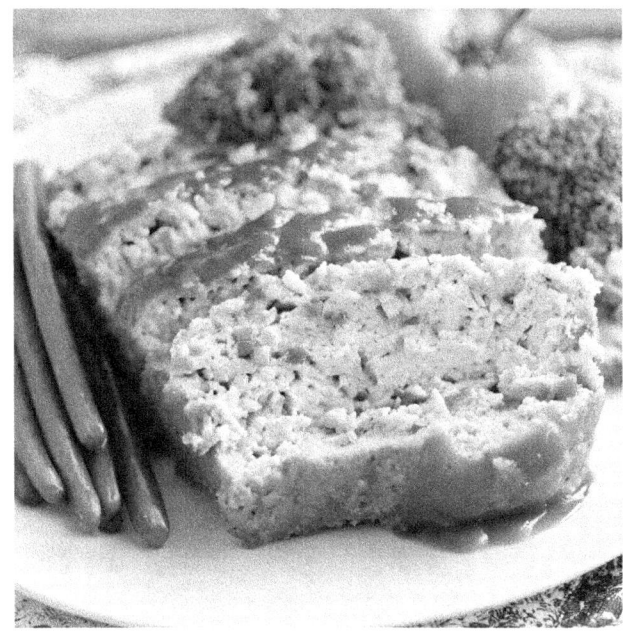

9. Smoked Turkey Breast

Ingredients

- 1 whole turkey breast (about 4-5 pounds), bone-in and skinless
- 1/4 cup olive oil
- 1/4 cup apple cider vinegar
- 1 tablespoon smoked paprika
- 1 tablespoon garlic powder
- 1 teaspoon dried thyme
- 1 teaspoon ground black pepper

Instructions

1. Preheat the smoker to 225°F (107°C).
2. In a small bowl, mix together olive oil, apple cider vinegar, smoked paprika, garlic powder, dried thyme, and ground black pepper.
3. Rub the mixture all over the turkey breast, ensuring it is evenly coated.
4. Place the turkey breast in the smoker.
5. Smoke the turkey for 3-4 hours, or until the internal temperature reaches 165°F (75°C).
6. Let the turkey rest for 10 minutes before slicing.
7. Serve hot.

Nutrition Info per Serving

- Calories: 250
- Carbohydrates: 2g
- Protein: 34g
- Fat: 12g
- Fiber: 0g
- Sodium: 100mg

Serves
8

Cooking Time
4 hours

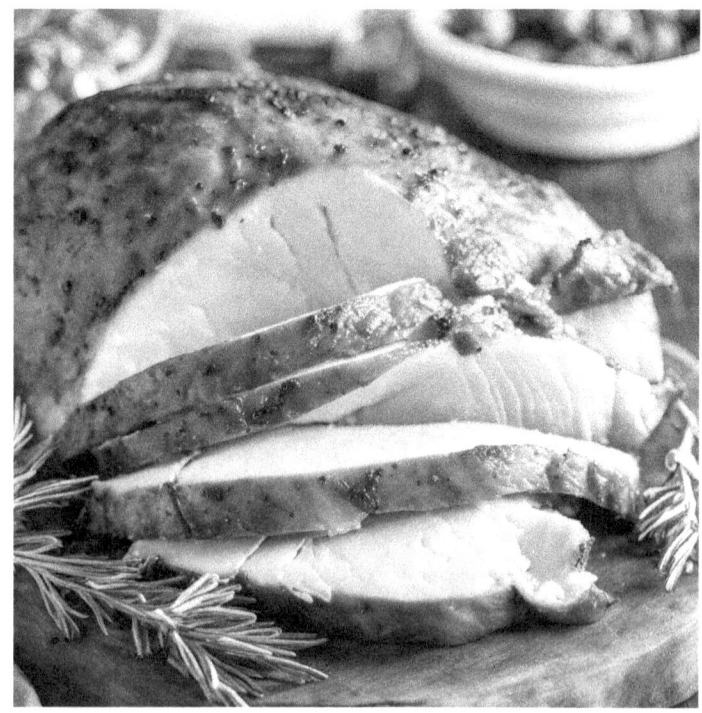

10. Turkey and Quinoa Stuffed Peppers

Ingredients

- 4 large bell peppers, tops cut off and seeds removed
- 1 pound ground turkey
- 1 cup cooked quinoa
- 1 cup diced tomatoes (canned, no salt added)
- 1/2 cup onion, finely chopped
- 1/2 cup black beans, drained and rinsed
- 1/2 cup corn kernels
- 2 garlic cloves, minced
- 1 teaspoon ground cumin
- 1 teaspoon paprika
- 1/2 teaspoon ground black pepper
- 1/2 cup shredded mozzarella cheese (optional)

Instructions

1. Preheat oven to 375°F (190°C).
2. In a large skillet, cook ground turkey over medium heat until browned, about 5-7 minutes.
3. Add onion and garlic to the skillet and cook for 3-4 minutes until softened.
4. Stir in diced tomatoes, black beans, corn, cooked quinoa, ground cumin, paprika, and ground black pepper. Cook for another 5 minutes until heated through.
5. Stuff each bell pepper with the turkey and quinoa mixture.
6. Place the stuffed peppers in a baking dish. If using, sprinkle shredded mozzarella cheese on top.
7. Cover with foil and bake for 25-30 minutes until peppers are tender.
8. Serve hot.

Nutrition Info per Serving

- Calories: 280
- Carbohydrates: 25g
- Protein: 28g
- Fat: 10g
- Fiber: 6g
- Sodium: 200mg

Serves

4

Cooking Time

40 minutes

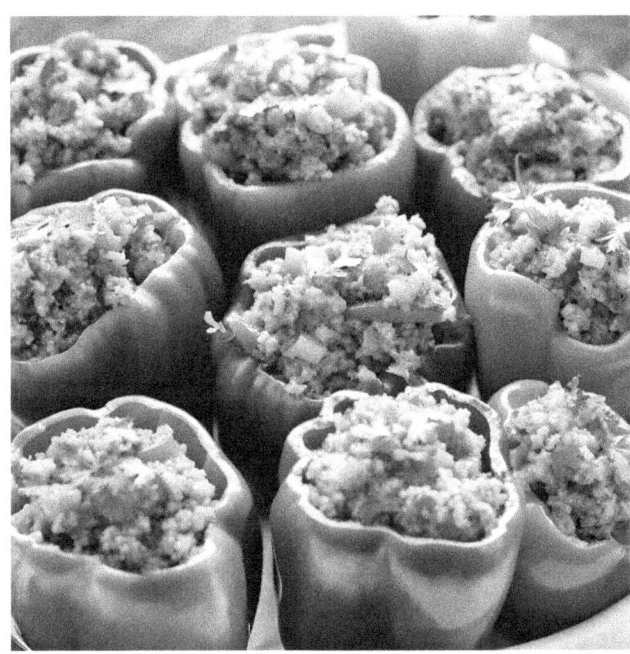

11. Turkey Bolognese

Ingredients

- 1 pound ground turkey
- 1 tablespoon olive oil
- 1 onion, finely chopped
- 3 garlic cloves, minced
- 1 carrot, grated
- 1 celery stalk, finely chopped
- 1 can (28 ounces) crushed tomatoes (no salt added)
- 1 teaspoon dried basil
- 1 teaspoon dried oregano
- 1/2 teaspoon ground black pepper
- 1/4 cup chopped fresh parsley
- 1/4 cup grated Parmesan cheese (optional)

Instructions

1. Heat olive oil in a large skillet over medium heat.
2. Add ground turkey and cook until browned, about 5-7 minutes.
3. Add onion, garlic, carrot, and celery. Cook for 5-7 minutes until vegetables are softened.
4. Stir in crushed tomatoes, dried basil, dried oregano, and ground black pepper. Bring to a simmer.
5. Reduce heat to low and let the sauce simmer for 30 minutes, stirring occasionally.
6. Stir in chopped fresh parsley and cook for another 5 minutes.
7. Serve hot, topped with grated Parmesan cheese if desired.

Nutrition Info per Serving

- Calories: 240
- Carbohydrates: 14g
- Protein: 28g
- Fat: 10g
- Fiber: 4g
- Sodium: 150mg

Serves

4

Cooking Time

45 minutes

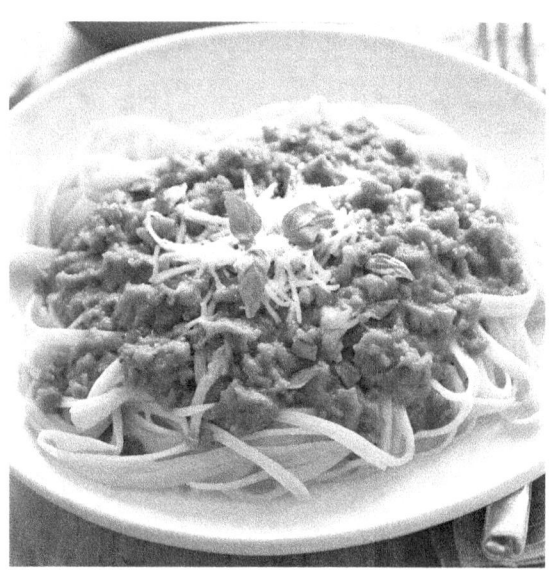

12. Turkey Skewers with Vegetables

Ingredients

- 1 pound turkey breast, cut into cubes
- 1 red bell pepper, cut into chunks
- 1 yellow bell pepper, cut into chunks
- 1 zucchini, sliced
- 1 red onion, cut into chunks
- 2 tablespoons olive oil
- 1 tablespoon lemon juice
- 1 teaspoon dried oregano
- 1 teaspoon ground black pepper
- Wooden skewers, soaked in water for 30 minutes

Instructions

1. In a large bowl, whisk together olive oil, lemon juice, dried oregano, and ground black pepper.
2. Add turkey cubes and vegetables to the bowl, tossing to coat well. Marinate for 30 minutes.
3. Preheat grill to medium-high heat.
4. Thread turkey and vegetables onto the skewers, alternating between turkey and vegetables.
5. Grill the skewers for 10-12 minutes, turning occasionally, until turkey is cooked through and vegetables are tender.
6. Serve hot.

Nutrition Info per Serving

- Calories: 220
- Carbohydrates: 8g
- Protein: 28g
- Fat: 10g
- Fiber: 3g
- Sodium: 100mg

Serves

4

Cooking Time

30 minutes (plus marinating time)

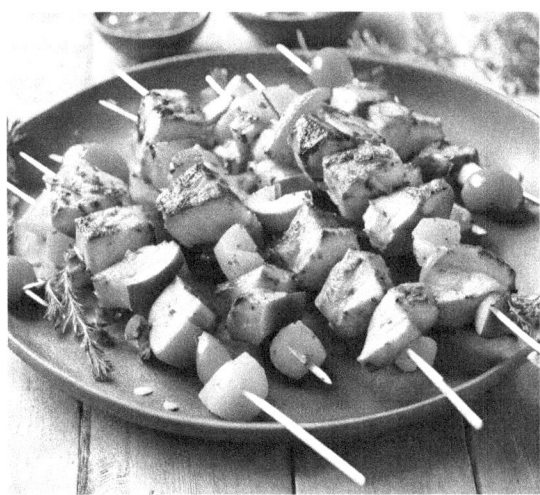

13. Creamy Turkey and Mushroom Soup
Ingredients
- 1 pound ground turkey
- 1 tablespoon olive oil
- 1 onion, chopped
- 2 garlic cloves, minced
- 2 cups mushrooms, sliced
- 1 carrot, chopped
- 2 celery stalks, chopped
- 4 cups low-sodium chicken broth
- 1 cup unsweetened almond milk
- 1 teaspoon dried thyme
- 1 teaspoon ground black pepper
- 2 tablespoons whole wheat flour
- 1/4 cup fresh parsley, chopped

Instructions
1. Heat olive oil in a large pot over medium heat.
2. Add ground turkey and cook until browned, about 5-7 minutes. Remove from pot and set aside.
3. In the same pot, add onion, garlic, mushrooms, carrot, and celery. Sauté for 5-7 minutes until vegetables are tender.
4. Stir in whole wheat flour and cook for 1 minute.
5. Add low-sodium chicken broth, almond milk, dried thyme, and ground black pepper. Bring to a boil.
6. Reduce heat and simmer for 20 minutes.
7. Return cooked turkey to the pot and cook for another 5 minutes.
8. Stir in chopped fresh parsley before serving.
9. Serve hot.

Nutrition Info per Serving
- Calories: 220
- Carbohydrates: 12g
- Protein: 28g
- Fat: 8g
- Fiber: 3g
- Sodium: 150mg

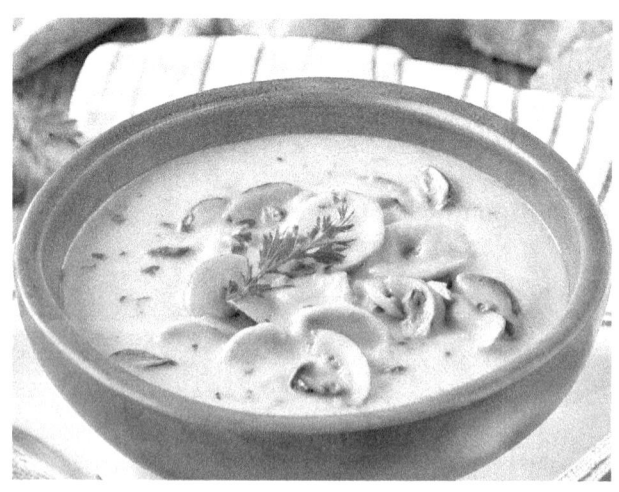

Serves
6
Cooking Time
35 minutes

14. Chicken and Turkey Sausage Jambalaya

Ingredients

- 1/2 pound boneless, skinless chicken breasts, cubed
- 1/2 pound turkey sausage, sliced
- 1 tablespoon olive oil
- 1 onion, chopped
- 3 garlic cloves, minced
- 1 green bell pepper, chopped
- 1 red bell pepper, chopped
- 1 cup brown rice
- 2 cups low-sodium chicken broth
- 1 can (14.5 ounces) diced tomatoes (no salt added)
- 1 teaspoon dried thyme
- 1 teaspoon smoked paprika
- 1/2 teaspoon ground black pepper
- 1/4 teaspoon cayenne pepper (optional)

Instructions

1. Heat olive oil in a large pot over medium heat.
2. Add cubed chicken and turkey sausage, cooking until browned, about 5-7 minutes.
3. Remove meat from the pot and set aside.
4. In the same pot, add onion, garlic, green bell pepper, and red bell pepper. Cook for 5-7 minutes until vegetables are tender.
5. Stir in brown rice, low-sodium chicken broth, diced tomatoes, dried thyme, smoked paprika, ground black pepper, and cayenne pepper if using. Bring to a boil.
6. Reduce heat, cover, and simmer for 30-35 minutes, until rice is tender and liquid is absorbed.
7. Return chicken and sausage to the pot, cooking for an additional 5 minutes until heated through.
8. Serve hot.

Nutrition Info per Serving

- Calories: 320
- Carbohydrates: 30g
- Protein: 28g
- Fat: 10g
- Fiber: 5g
- Sodium: 300mg

Serves

6

Cooking Time

45 minutes

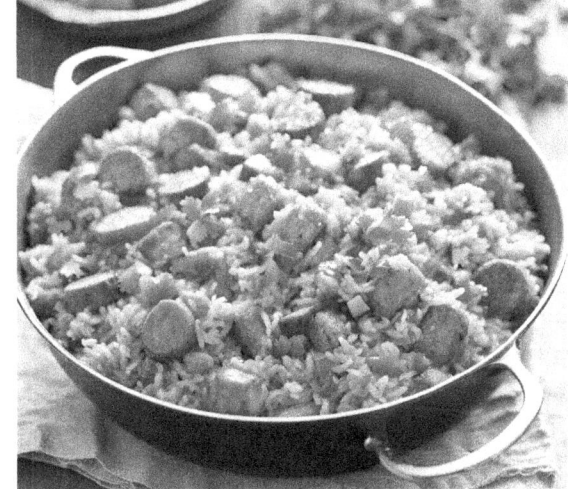

15. Poultry Shepherd's Pie

Ingredients

- 1 pound ground turkey
- 1 pound ground chicken
- 1 tablespoon olive oil
- 1 onion, finely chopped
- 3 garlic cloves, minced
- 2 carrots, diced
- 1 cup peas (fresh or frozen)
- 1 cup corn (fresh or frozen)
- 1 tablespoon tomato paste
- 1 cup low-sodium chicken broth
- 1 teaspoon dried thyme
- 1 teaspoon ground black pepper
- 4 cups mashed potatoes (prepared with unsweetened almond milk and olive oil)

Instructions

1. Preheat oven to 375°F (190°C).
2. Heat olive oil in a large skillet over medium heat. Add onion and garlic, sautéing until softened, about 3-4 minutes.
3. Add ground turkey and chicken, cooking until browned, about 5-7 minutes.
4. Stir in carrots, peas, corn, tomato paste, chicken broth, dried thyme, and ground black pepper. Simmer for 10 minutes, until vegetables are tender and the mixture thickens.
5. Transfer the meat mixture to a baking dish and spread evenly.
6. Top with mashed potatoes, spreading them evenly over the meat mixture.
7. Bake for 25-30 minutes, until the top is golden brown.
8. Serve hot.

Nutrition Info per Serving

- Calories: 320
- Carbohydrates: 28g
- Protein: 30g
- Fat: 12g
- Fiber: 5g
- Sodium: 200mg

Serves
6

Cooking Time
45 minutes

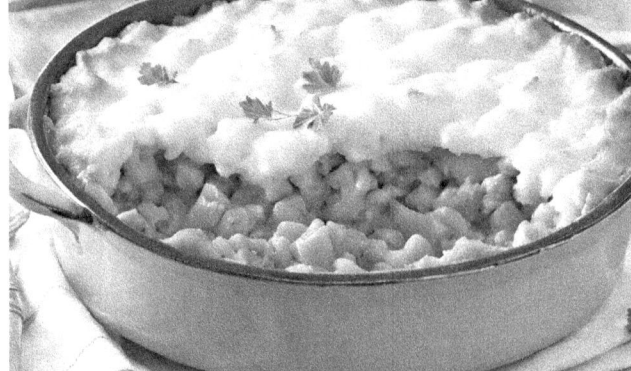

16. BBQ Pulled Chicken

Ingredients

- 4 boneless, skinless chicken breasts
- 1 cup low-sugar BBQ sauce
- 1/2 cup apple cider vinegar
- 1 tablespoon olive oil
- 1 teaspoon ground black pepper
- 1 teaspoon smoked paprika
- 1/2 teaspoon garlic powder

Instructions

1. Place chicken breasts in a slow cooker.
2. In a bowl, mix together BBQ sauce, apple cider vinegar, olive oil, ground black pepper, smoked paprika, and garlic powder.
3. Pour the mixture over the chicken breasts.
4. Cover and cook on low for 6-7 hours, or until the chicken is tender and easily shredded.
5. Shred the chicken with two forks and stir to coat with the sauce.
6. Serve hot.

Nutrition Info per Serving

- Calories: 250
- Carbohydrates: 10g
- Protein: 30g
- Fat: 10g
- Fiber: 2g
- Sodium: 300mg

Serves

4

Cooking Time

7 hours

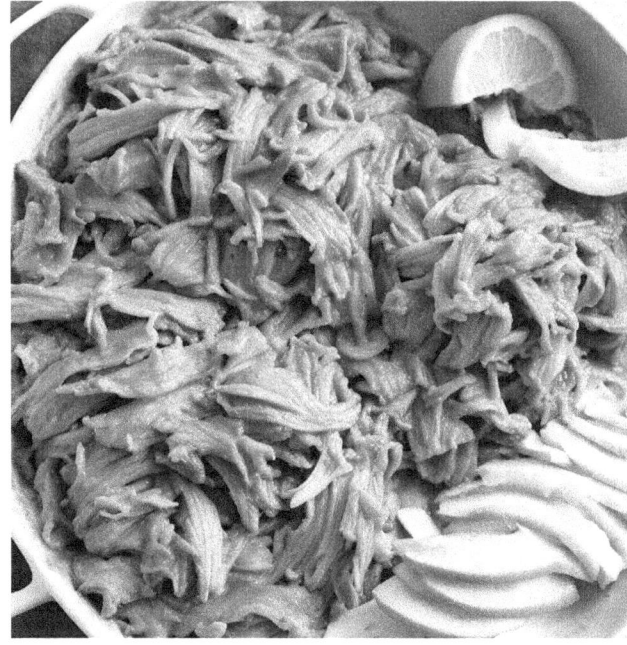

17. Chicken and Turkey Meatballs

Ingredients

- 1/2 pound ground turkey
- 1/2 pound ground chicken
- 1/4 cup whole wheat breadcrumbs
- 1/4 cup grated Parmesan cheese
- 1 egg, beaten
- 2 garlic cloves, minced
- 1 teaspoon dried oregano
- 1 teaspoon ground black pepper
- 1 tablespoon olive oil

Instructions

1. Preheat oven to 375°F (190°C).
2. In a large bowl, combine ground turkey, ground chicken, whole wheat breadcrumbs, grated Parmesan cheese, beaten egg, minced garlic, dried oregano, and ground black pepper. Mix until well combined.
3. Form the mixture into 1-inch meatballs and place on a baking sheet lined with parchment paper.
4. Heat olive oil in a large skillet over medium heat. Brown the meatballs for 2-3 minutes on each side.
5. Transfer the meatballs to the preheated oven and bake for 15-20 minutes, until cooked through.
6. Serve hot.

Nutrition Info per Serving

- Calories: 220
- Carbohydrates: 6g
- Protein: 26g
- Fat: 10g
- Fiber: 1g
- Sodium: 200mg

Serves

4

Cooking Time

30 minutes

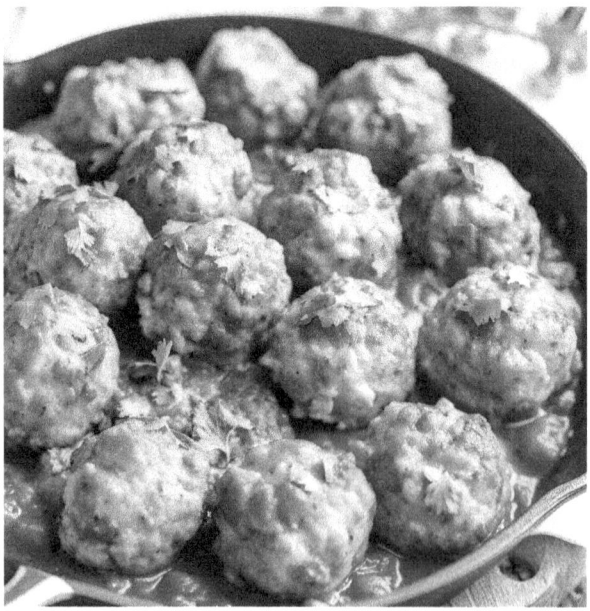

18. Turkey Broth Soup with Kale

Ingredients

- 1 pound ground turkey
- 1 tablespoon olive oil
- 1 onion, chopped
- 3 garlic cloves, minced
- 2 carrots, sliced
- 2 celery stalks, sliced
- 6 cups low-sodium chicken broth
- 2 cups chopped kale
- 1 teaspoon dried thyme
- 1 teaspoon ground black pepper
- 1/2 cup quinoa, rinsed

Instructions

1. Heat olive oil in a large pot over medium heat. Add ground turkey and cook until browned, about 5-7 minutes.
2. Add chopped onion, minced garlic, sliced carrots, and sliced celery. Cook for 5-7 minutes until vegetables are tender.
3. Stir in low-sodium chicken broth, chopped kale, dried thyme, ground black pepper, and quinoa. Bring to a boil.
4. Reduce heat and simmer for 20-25 minutes, until quinoa is tender.
5. Serve hot.

Nutrition Info per Serving

- Calories: 220
- Carbohydrates: 18g
- Protein: 28g
- Fat: 8g
- Fiber: 5g
- Sodium: 150mg

Serves
6

Cooking Time
35 minutes

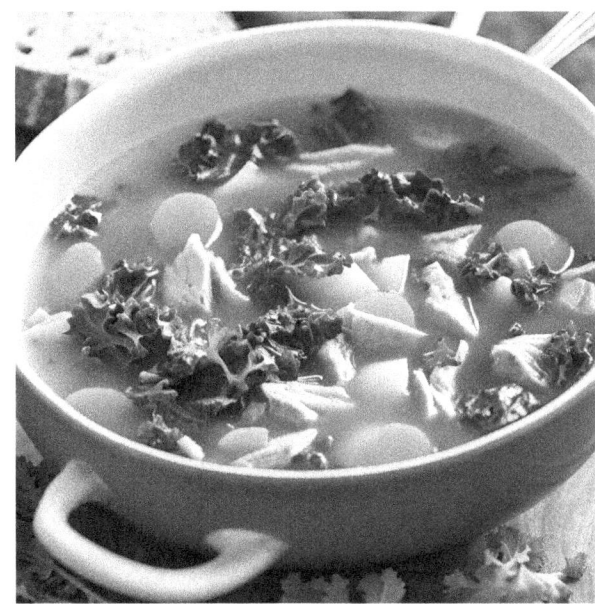

19. Turkey Piccata

Ingredients

- 4 turkey cutlets (about 1 pound)
- 1/4 cup whole wheat flour
- 2 tablespoons olive oil
- 1/4 cup lemon juice
- 1/4 cup low-sodium chicken broth
- 2 tablespoons capers, rinsed and drained
- 1 teaspoon ground black pepper
- 2 tablespoons chopped fresh parsley

Instructions

1. Dredge turkey cutlets in whole wheat flour, shaking off excess.
2. Heat olive oil in a large skillet over medium-high heat. Add turkey cutlets and cook for 2-3 minutes on each side, until golden brown and cooked through. Remove from skillet and set aside.
3. In the same skillet, add lemon juice, low-sodium chicken broth, capers, and ground black pepper. Cook for 2-3 minutes, stirring to combine and scrape up any browned bits from the bottom of the skillet.
4. Return turkey cutlets to the skillet, spooning sauce over the top. Cook for an additional 2 minutes until heated through.
5. Sprinkle with chopped fresh parsley before serving.
6. Serve hot.

Nutrition Info per Serving

- Calories: 240
- Carbohydrates: 8g
- Protein: 30g
- Fat: 10g
- Fiber: 1g
- Sodium: 150mg

Serves

4

Cooking Time

20 minutes

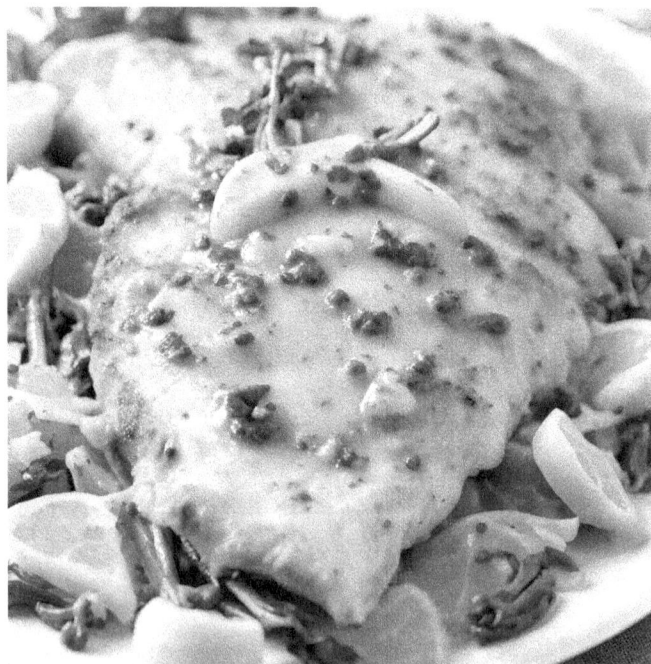

20. Poached Chicken Salad

Ingredients

- 2 boneless, skinless chicken breasts
- 4 cups low-sodium chicken broth
- 1 bay leaf
- 1 teaspoon dried thyme
- 4 cups mixed greens (spinach, arugula, lettuce)
- 1/2 cup cherry tomatoes, halved
- 1/4 cup red onion, thinly sliced
- 1/4 cup cucumber, sliced
- 1/4 cup feta cheese, crumbled
- 2 tablespoons olive oil
- 1 tablespoon balsamic vinegar
- 1 teaspoon Dijon mustard

Instructions

1. In a large pot, bring the chicken broth to a simmer with the bay leaf and dried thyme.
2. Add the chicken breasts and poach for 15-20 minutes until fully cooked.
3. Remove the chicken from the pot and let it cool. Once cooled, shred the chicken.
4. In a large bowl, combine mixed greens, cherry tomatoes, red onion, cucumber, and feta cheese.
5. In a small bowl, whisk together olive oil, balsamic vinegar, and Dijon mustard.
6. Toss the salad with the dressing and top with shredded chicken.
7. Serve immediately.

Nutrition Info per Serving

- Calories: 250
- Carbohydrates: 8g
- Protein: 30g
- Fat: 12g
- Fiber: 2g
- Sodium: 150mg

Serves
4
Cooking Time
30 minutes

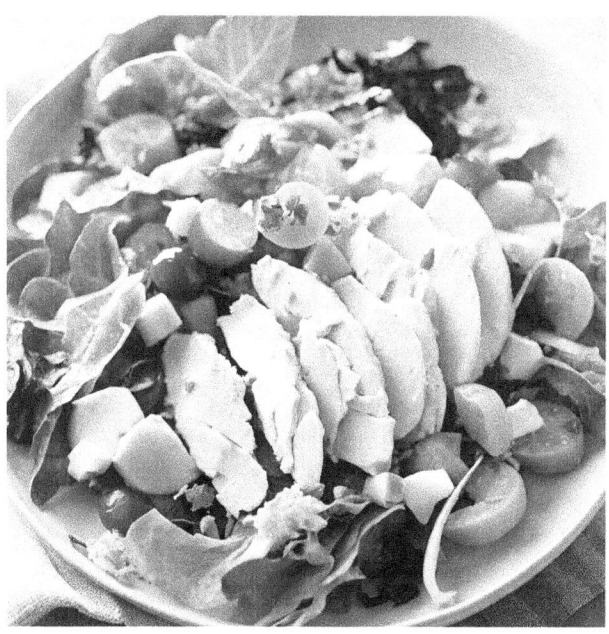

21. Turkey and Cranberry Sliders

Ingredients

- 1 pound ground turkey
- 1/2 cup whole wheat breadcrumbs
- 1 egg, beaten
- 2 garlic cloves, minced
- 1 teaspoon dried sage
- 1 teaspoon ground black pepper
- 1/4 cup cranberry sauce (low sugar)
- 8 whole wheat slider buns
- 1/4 cup mixed greens

Instructions

1. Preheat oven to 375°F (190°C).
2. In a large bowl, combine ground turkey, whole wheat breadcrumbs, beaten egg, minced garlic, dried sage, and ground black pepper. Mix until well combined.
3. Form the mixture into 8 small patties and place them on a baking sheet lined with parchment paper.
4. Bake for 15-20 minutes, or until fully cooked.
5. Assemble the sliders by placing each turkey patty on a whole wheat bun, topping with cranberry sauce and mixed greens.
6. Serve immediately.

Nutrition Info per Serving

- Calories: 240
- Carbohydrates: 24g
- Protein: 22g
- Fat: 8g
- Fiber: 3g
- Sodium: 180mg

Serves
8 sliders
Cooking Time
30 minutes

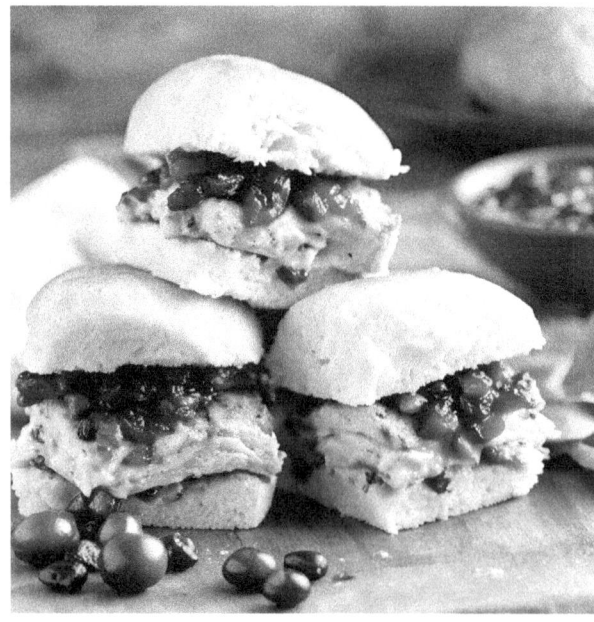

22. Chicken Paella with Brown Rice
Ingredients
- 1 pound boneless, skinless chicken thighs, cut into pieces
- 1 tablespoon olive oil
- 1 onion, chopped
- 3 garlic cloves, minced
- 1 red bell pepper, chopped
- 1 yellow bell pepper, chopped
- 1 cup brown rice
- 2 cups low-sodium chicken broth
- 1 can (14.5 ounces) diced tomatoes (no salt added)
- 1 teaspoon smoked paprika
- 1/2 teaspoon ground turmeric
- 1/2 teaspoon ground black pepper
- 1 cup peas (fresh or frozen)
- 1/4 cup chopped fresh parsley

Instructions
1. Heat olive oil in a large skillet or paella pan over medium heat.
2. Add the chicken pieces and cook until browned, about 5-7 minutes. Remove from the skillet and set aside.
3. In the same skillet, add onion, garlic, and bell peppers. Cook for 5-7 minutes until vegetables are tender.
4. Stir in the brown rice, chicken broth, diced tomatoes, smoked paprika, ground turmeric, and ground black pepper. Bring to a boil.
5. Reduce heat, cover, and simmer for 35-40 minutes until the rice is tender and liquid is absorbed.
6. Stir in the peas and cooked chicken, cooking for an additional 5 minutes until heated through.
7. Sprinkle with chopped fresh parsley before serving.
8. Serve hot.

Nutrition Info per Serving
- Calories: 320
- Carbohydrates: 38g
- Protein: 28g
- Fat: 8g
- Fiber: 5g
- Sodium: 200mg

Serves
6
Cooking Time
50 minutes

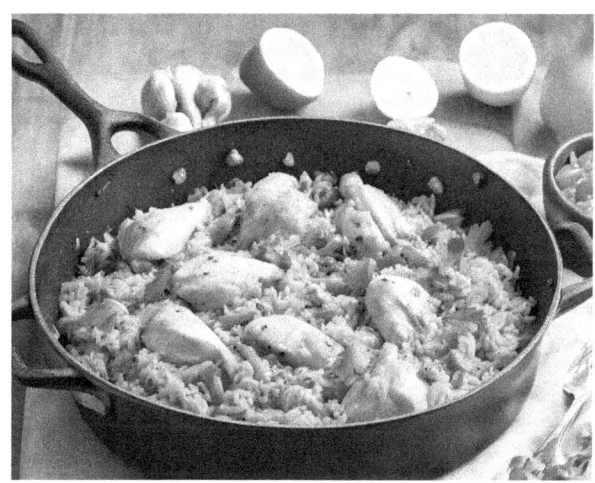

23. Turkey and Spinach Meatballs

Ingredients

- 1 pound ground turkey
- 1 cup fresh spinach, finely chopped
- 1/4 cup whole wheat breadcrumbs
- 1 egg, beaten
- 2 garlic cloves, minced
- 1 teaspoon dried oregano
- 1 teaspoon ground black pepper
- 1 tablespoon olive oil

Instructions

1. Preheat oven to 375°F (190°C).
2. In a large bowl, combine ground turkey, chopped spinach, whole wheat breadcrumbs, beaten egg, minced garlic, dried oregano, and ground black pepper. Mix until well combined.
3. Form the mixture into 1-inch meatballs and place them on a baking sheet lined with parchment paper.
4. Heat olive oil in a large skillet over medium heat. Brown the meatballs for 2-3 minutes on each side.
5. Transfer the meatballs to the preheated oven and bake for 15-20 minutes, until cooked through.
6. Serve hot.

Nutrition Info per Serving

- Calories: 210
- Carbohydrates: 5g
- Protein: 25g
- Fat: 10g
- Fiber: 1g
- Sodium: 150mg

Serves

4

Cooking Time

30 minutes

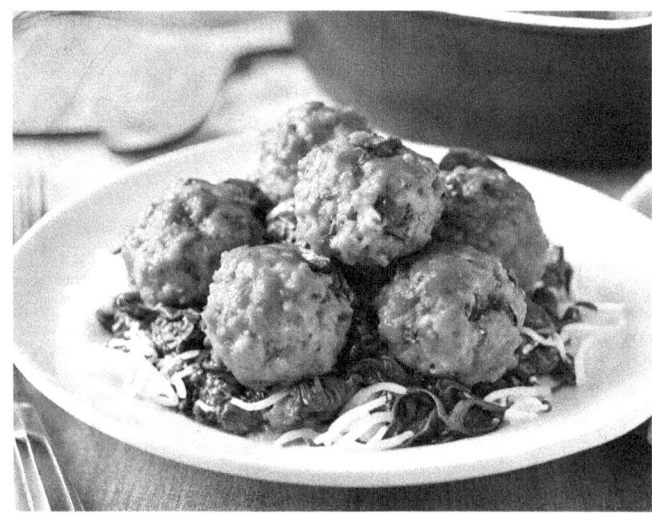

24. Turkey Pot Pie

Ingredients

- 1 pound ground turkey
- 1 tablespoon olive oil
- 1 onion, chopped
- 3 garlic cloves, minced
- 2 carrots, diced
- 1 cup peas (fresh or frozen)
- 1 cup corn (fresh or frozen)
- 2 cups low-sodium chicken broth
- 1/2 cup unsweetened almond milk
- 1 teaspoon dried thyme
- 1 teaspoon ground black pepper
- 2 tablespoons whole wheat flour
- 1 whole wheat pie crust

Instructions

1. Preheat oven to 375°F (190°C).
2. Heat olive oil in a large skillet over medium heat. Add ground turkey and cook until browned, about 5-7 minutes.
3. Add onion, garlic, carrots, peas, and corn. Cook for 5-7 minutes until vegetables are tender.
4. Stir in the whole wheat flour and cook for 1 minute.
5. Add chicken broth, almond milk, dried thyme, and ground black pepper. Bring to a simmer and cook until thickened, about 5 minutes.
6. Transfer the mixture to a baking dish and cover with the whole wheat pie crust.
7. Bake for 25-30 minutes, until the crust is golden brown.
8. Serve hot.

Nutrition Info per Serving

- Calories: 300
- Carbohydrates: 30g
- Protein: 25g
- Fat: 12g
- Fiber: 4g
- Sodium: 200mg

Serves

6

Cooking Time

45 minutes

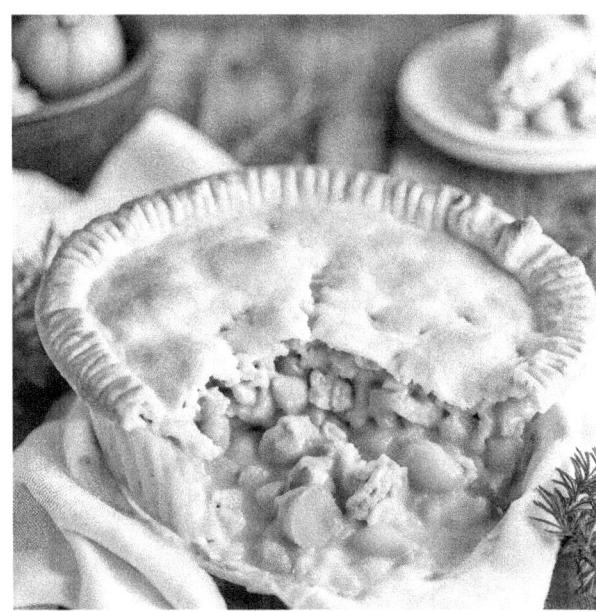

25. Turkey Noodle Soup

Ingredients

- 1 pound ground turkey
- 1 tablespoon olive oil
- 1 onion, chopped
- 3 garlic cloves, minced
- 2 carrots, sliced
- 2 celery stalks, sliced
- 6 cups low-sodium chicken broth
- 1 cup whole wheat egg noodles
- 1 teaspoon dried thyme
- 1 teaspoon ground black pepper
- 2 cups fresh spinach, chopped

Instructions

1. Heat olive oil in a large pot over medium heat. Add ground turkey and cook until browned, about 5-7 minutes.
2. Add chopped onion, minced garlic, sliced carrots, and sliced celery. Cook for 5-7 minutes until vegetables are tender.
3. Stir in low-sodium chicken broth, whole wheat egg noodles, dried thyme, and ground black pepper. Bring to a boil.
4. Reduce heat and simmer for 15 minutes, until noodles are tender.
5. Stir in chopped spinach and cook for an additional 5 minutes.
6. Serve hot.

Nutrition Info per Serving

- Calories: 230
- Carbohydrates: 18g
- Protein: 26g
- Fat: 8g
- Fiber: 4g
- Sodium: 150mg

Serves

6

Cooking Time

35 minutes

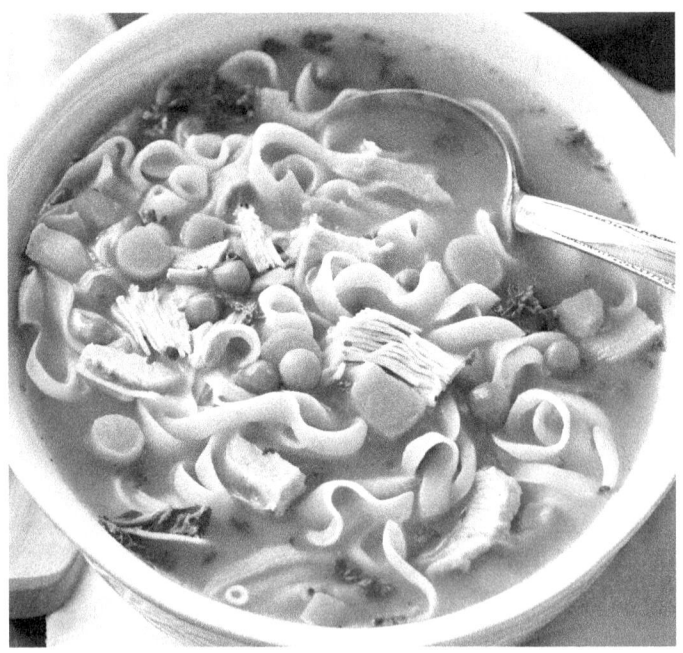

Fish & Seafood Recipes

1. Grilled Salmon with Dill
Ingredients
- 4 salmon fillets (about 6 ounces each)
- 2 tablespoons olive oil
- 2 tablespoons fresh lemon juice
- 2 tablespoons fresh dill, chopped
- 3 garlic cloves, minced
- 1 teaspoon ground black pepper

Instructions
1. Preheat the grill to medium-high heat.
2. In a small bowl, whisk together olive oil, lemon juice, chopped dill, minced garlic, and ground black pepper.
3. Brush the mixture over the salmon fillets.
4. Grill the salmon for 4-5 minutes on each side, or until the fish is cooked through and flakes easily with a fork.
5. Serve hot.

Nutrition Info per Serving
- Calories: 310
- Carbohydrates: 2g
- Protein: 34g
- Fat: 18g
- Fiber: 0g
- Sodium: 75mg

Serves
4
Cooking Time
10 minutes

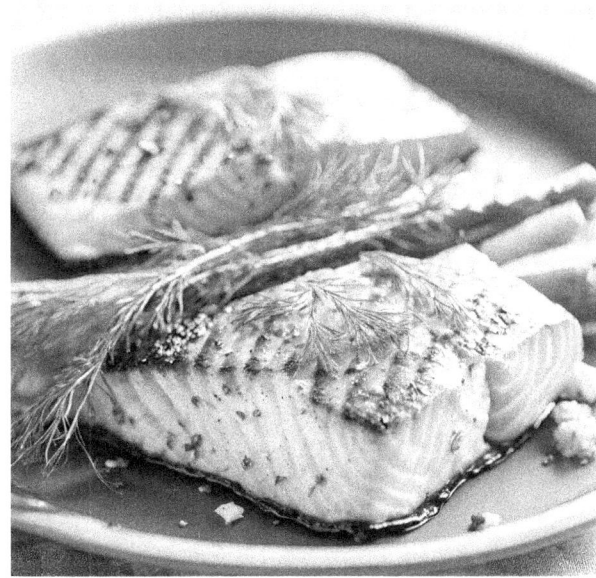

2. Baked Cod with Lemon and Capers

Ingredients

- 4 cod fillets (about 6 ounces each)
- 2 tablespoons olive oil
- 2 tablespoons fresh lemon juice
- 2 tablespoons capers, rinsed and drained
- 1 teaspoon dried oregano
- 1 teaspoon ground black pepper

Instructions

1. Preheat the oven to 375°F (190°C).
2. Place the cod fillets in a baking dish.
3. In a small bowl, whisk together olive oil, lemon juice, capers, dried oregano, and ground black pepper.
4. Pour the mixture over the cod fillets.
5. Bake for 15-20 minutes, or until the fish is cooked through and flakes easily with a fork.
6. Serve hot.

Nutrition Info per Serving

- Calories: 220
- Carbohydrates: 2g
- Protein: 34g
- Fat: 8g
- Fiber: 0g
- Sodium: 170mg

Serves

4

Cooking Time

20 minutes

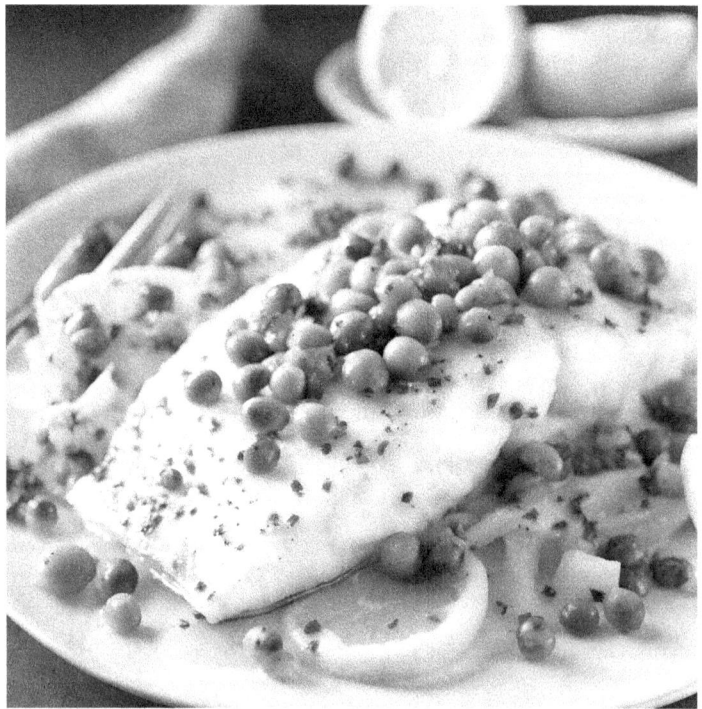

3. Tilapia Piccata

Ingredients

- 4 tilapia fillets (about 6 ounces each)
- 1/4 cup whole wheat flour
- 2 tablespoons olive oil
- 1/4 cup fresh lemon juice
- 1/4 cup low-sodium chicken broth
- 2 tablespoons capers, rinsed and drained
- 1 teaspoon ground black pepper
- 2 tablespoons fresh parsley, chopped

Instructions

1. Dredge tilapia fillets in whole wheat flour, shaking off excess.
2. Heat olive oil in a large skillet over medium-high heat. Add tilapia fillets and cook for 3-4 minutes on each side, until golden brown and cooked through. Remove from the skillet and set aside.
3. In the same skillet, add lemon juice, chicken broth, capers, and ground black pepper. Cook for 2-3 minutes, stirring to combine.
4. Return tilapia fillets to the skillet, spooning sauce over the top. Cook for an additional 2 minutes until heated through.
5. Sprinkle with chopped parsley before serving.
6. Serve hot.

Nutrition Info per Serving

- Calories: 240
- Carbohydrates: 8g
- Protein: 32g
- Fat: 10g
- Fiber: 1g
- Sodium: 150mg

Serves

4

Cooking Time

20 minutes

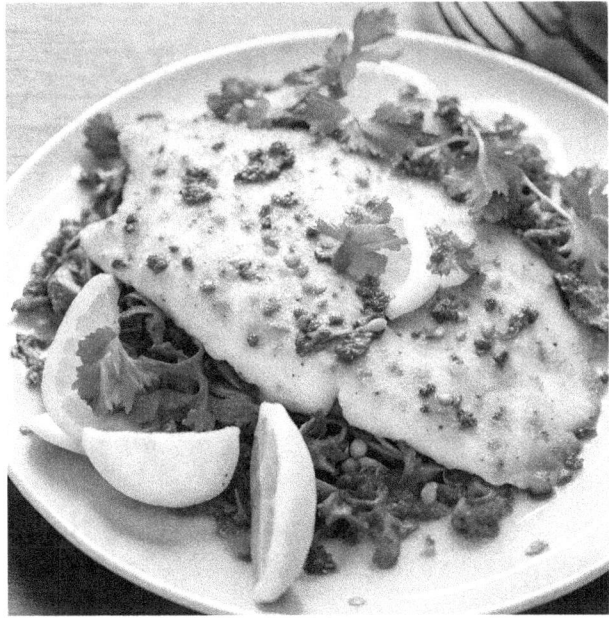

4. Herb-Crusted Halibut

Ingredients

- 4 halibut fillets (about 6 ounces each)
- 1/2 cup whole wheat breadcrumbs
- 1/4 cup grated Parmesan cheese
- 2 tablespoons fresh parsley, chopped
- 1 tablespoon fresh thyme, chopped
- 3 garlic cloves, minced
- 1 tablespoon olive oil
- 1 teaspoon ground black pepper

Instructions

1. Preheat the oven to 400°F (200°C).
2. In a small bowl, combine whole wheat breadcrumbs, grated Parmesan cheese, chopped parsley, chopped thyme, minced garlic, olive oil, and ground black pepper.
3. Press the breadcrumb mixture onto the top of each halibut fillet.
4. Place the halibut fillets on a baking sheet lined with parchment paper.
5. Bake for 12-15 minutes, or until the fish is cooked through and the crust is golden brown.
6. Serve hot.

Nutrition Info per Serving

- Calories: 280
- Carbohydrates: 10g
- Protein: 36g
- Fat: 12g
- Fiber: 1g
- Sodium: 200mg

Serves

4

Cooking Time

15 minutes

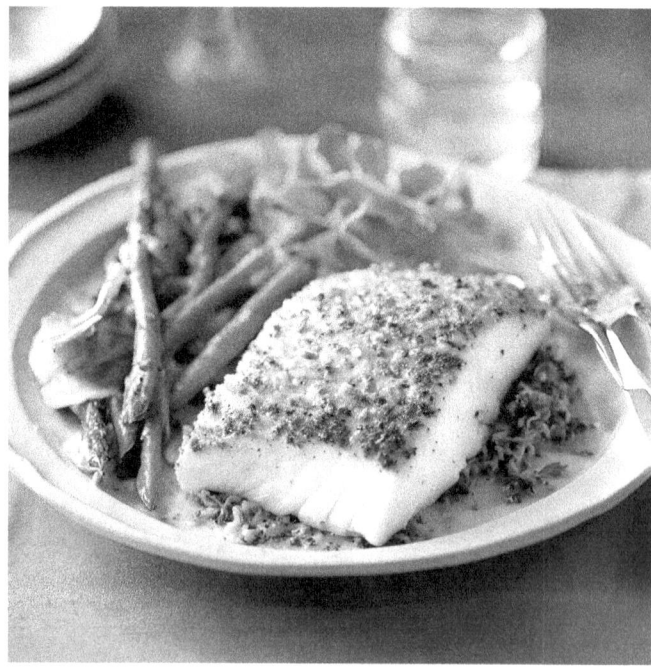

5. Asian-Style Tuna Steaks

Ingredients

- 4 tuna steaks (about 6 ounces each)
- 1/4 cup low-sodium soy sauce
- 2 tablespoons sesame oil
- 2 tablespoons rice vinegar
- 2 tablespoons honey
- 1 tablespoon fresh ginger, grated
- 2 garlic cloves, minced
- 1 tablespoon sesame seeds
- 2 green onions, thinly sliced

Instructions

1. In a small bowl, whisk together soy sauce, sesame oil, rice vinegar, honey, grated ginger, and minced garlic.
2. Place the tuna steaks in a shallow dish and pour the marinade over them. Let marinate for 15-20 minutes.
3. Preheat a grill or grill pan over medium-high heat.
4. Remove the tuna steaks from the marinade and discard the marinade.
5. Grill the tuna steaks for 2-3 minutes on each side, until desired doneness.
6. Sprinkle with sesame seeds and green onions before serving.
7. Serve hot.

Nutrition Info per Serving

- Calories: 300
- Carbohydrates: 8g
- Protein: 38g
- Fat: 12g
- Fiber: 1g
- Sodium: 300mg

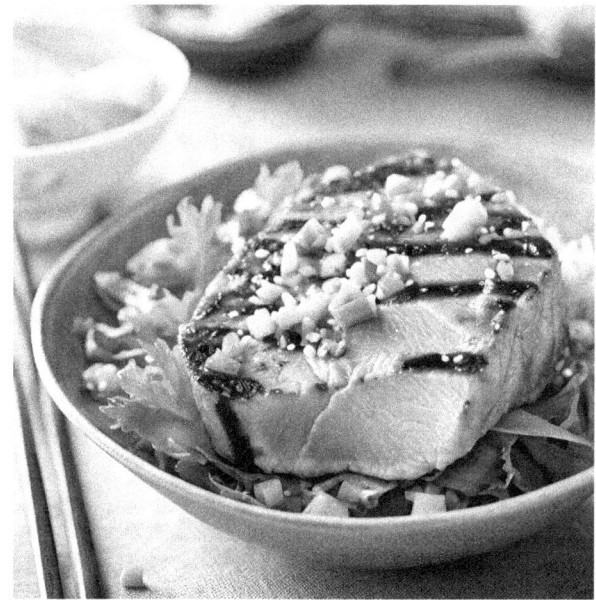

Serves

4

Cooking Time

20 minutes (plus marinating time)

6. Poached Salmon with Asparagus

Ingredients

- 4 salmon fillets (about 6 ounces each)
- 4 cups low-sodium vegetable broth
- 1 lemon, sliced
- 1 bay leaf
- 1 bunch asparagus, trimmed
- 2 tablespoons olive oil
- 1 teaspoon ground black pepper
- 2 tablespoons fresh dill, chopped

Instructions

1. In a large skillet, bring the vegetable broth, lemon slices, and bay leaf to a simmer.
2. Add the salmon fillets and poach for 8-10 minutes, until the salmon is cooked through.
3. Meanwhile, steam the asparagus until tender, about 5-7 minutes.
4. Remove the salmon from the skillet and set aside.
5. Drizzle the asparagus with olive oil and sprinkle with ground black pepper.
6. Serve the poached salmon with steamed asparagus, garnished with chopped dill.
7. Serve hot.

Nutrition Info per Serving

- Calories: 310
- Carbohydrates: 6g
- Protein: 34g
- Fat: 18g
- Fiber: 3g
- Sodium: 120mg

Serves
4
Cooking Time
20 minutes

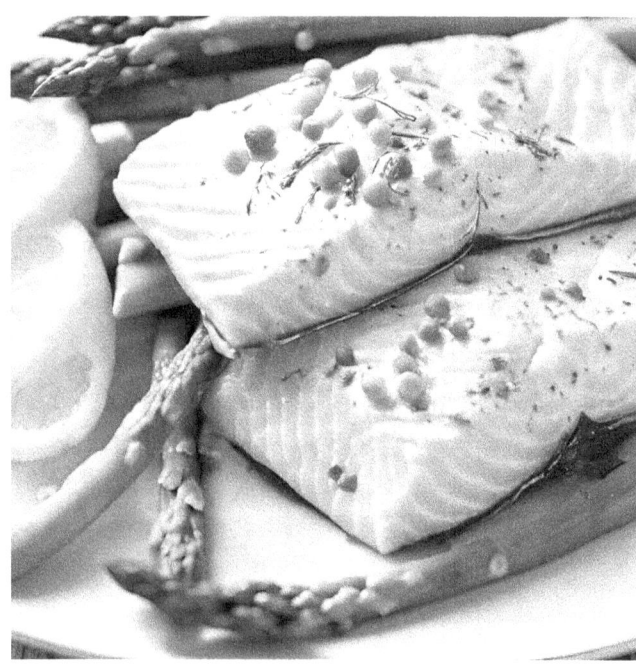

7. Smoked Haddock Chowder

Ingredients

- 1 pound smoked haddock fillets
- 1 tablespoon olive oil
- 1 onion, chopped
- 2 garlic cloves, minced
- 2 potatoes, peeled and diced
- 2 carrots, diced
- 4 cups low-sodium vegetable broth
- 1 cup unsweetened almond milk
- 1 teaspoon dried thyme
- 1 teaspoon ground black pepper
- 1/4 cup fresh parsley, chopped

Instructions

1. Heat olive oil in a large pot over medium heat. Add chopped onion and minced garlic, cooking for 3-4 minutes until softened.
2. Add diced potatoes and carrots, cooking for another 5 minutes.
3. Pour in the vegetable broth and bring to a boil. Reduce heat and simmer for 15 minutes, until vegetables are tender.
4. Add the smoked haddock fillets and cook for another 10 minutes until the fish is cooked through.
5. Stir in the almond milk, dried thyme, and ground black pepper. Simmer for another 5 minutes.
6. Remove from heat and gently flake the haddock into the chowder.
7. Sprinkle with fresh parsley before serving.
8. Serve hot.

Nutrition Info per Serving

- Calories: 250
- Carbohydrates: 20g
- Protein: 28g
- Fat: 8g
- Fiber: 4g
- Sodium: 200mg

Serves

4

Cooking Time

35 minutes

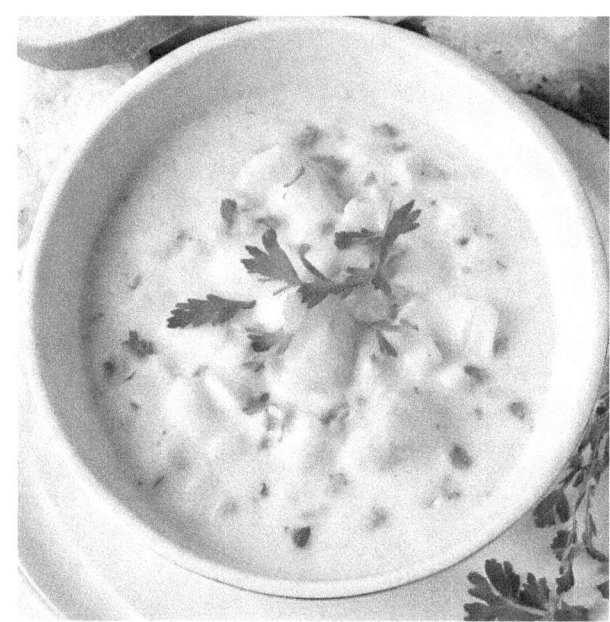

8. Mackerel with Tomato Salad

Ingredients

- 4 mackerel fillets (about 6 ounces each)
- 2 tablespoons olive oil
- 1 teaspoon ground black pepper
- 2 cups cherry tomatoes, halved
- 1/4 cup red onion, thinly sliced
- 1/4 cup fresh basil, chopped
- 2 tablespoons balsamic vinegar

Instructions

1. Preheat the grill to medium-high heat.
2. Brush the mackerel fillets with olive oil and sprinkle with ground black pepper.
3. Grill the mackerel for 4-5 minutes on each side, until the fish is cooked through and flakes easily with a fork.
4. In a bowl, combine halved cherry tomatoes, thinly sliced red onion, chopped basil, and balsamic vinegar.
5. Serve the grilled mackerel with the tomato salad on the side.
6. Serve hot.

Nutrition Info per Serving

- Calories: 320
- Carbohydrates: 8g
- Protein: 30g
- Fat: 20g
- Fiber: 2g
- Sodium: 120mg

Serves

4

Cooking Time

15 minutes

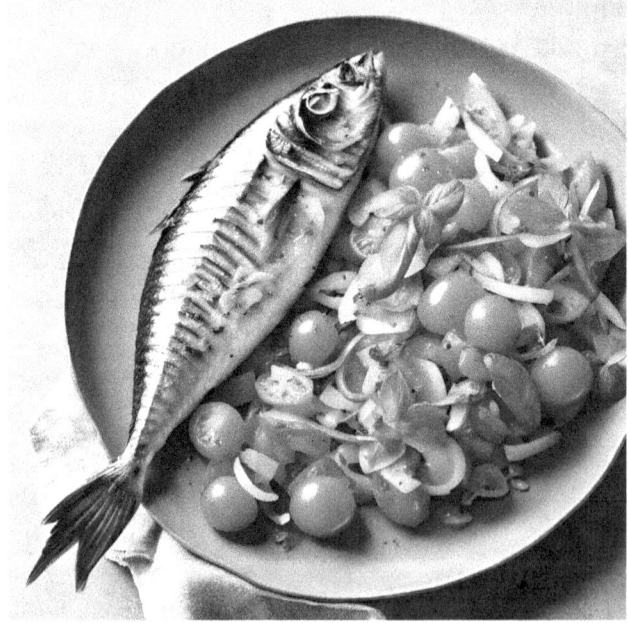

9. Trout Almondine
Ingredients
- 4 trout fillets (about 6 ounces each)
- 1/4 cup whole wheat flour
- 1/4 cup sliced almonds
- 3 tablespoons olive oil
- 1/4 cup fresh lemon juice
- 2 tablespoons fresh parsley, chopped
- 1 teaspoon ground black pepper

Instructions
1. Dredge the trout fillets in whole wheat flour, shaking off excess.
2. Heat 2 tablespoons of olive oil in a large skillet over medium heat. Add the trout fillets and cook for 4-5 minutes on each side, until golden brown and cooked through. Remove from the skillet and set aside.
3. In the same skillet, add the remaining olive oil and sliced almonds. Cook until the almonds are golden brown, about 2-3 minutes.
4. Stir in the lemon juice and ground black pepper.
5. Pour the almond and lemon mixture over the trout fillets.
6. Garnish with fresh parsley before serving.
7. Serve hot.

Nutrition Info per Serving
- Calories: 300
- Carbohydrates: 6g
- Protein: 32g
- Fat: 16g
- Fiber: 2g
- Sodium: 70mg

Serves
4
Cooking Time
15 minutes

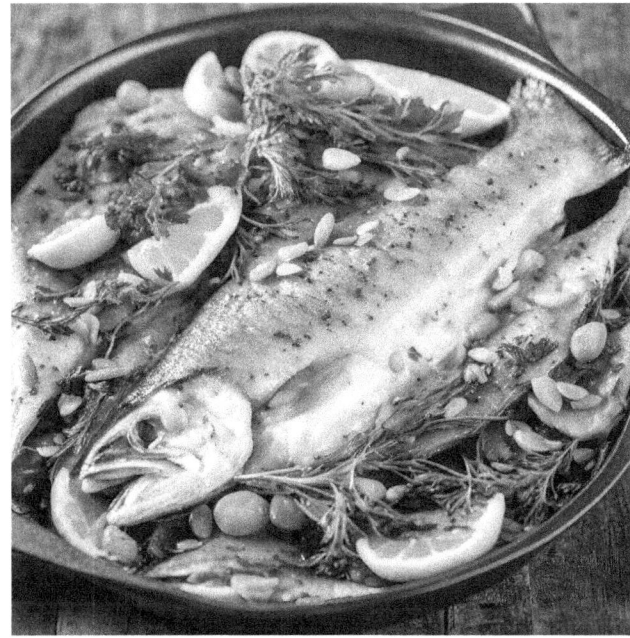

10. Shrimp Stir-Fry with Vegetables

Ingredients

- 1 pound shrimp, peeled and deveined
- 2 tablespoons olive oil
- 1 red bell pepper, sliced
- 1 yellow bell pepper, sliced
- 1 cup broccoli florets
- 1 carrot, julienned
- 1 cup snap peas
- 3 garlic cloves, minced
- 1 tablespoon grated ginger
- 1/4 cup low-sodium soy sauce
- 1 tablespoon rice vinegar
- 1 tablespoon honey
- 1 teaspoon ground black pepper

Instructions

1. In a small bowl, whisk together soy sauce, rice vinegar, honey, and ground black pepper. Set aside.
2. Heat olive oil in a large skillet or wok over medium-high heat.
3. Add shrimp and cook until pink, about 3-4 minutes. Remove shrimp from the skillet and set aside.
4. In the same skillet, add garlic and ginger. Sauté for 1 minute.
5. Add bell peppers, broccoli, carrot, and snap peas. Stir-fry for about 5-7 minutes, until vegetables are tender-crisp.
6. Return the shrimp to the skillet and pour the soy sauce mixture over the top. Stir to combine and cook for another 2 minutes.
7. Serve hot.

Nutrition Info per Serving

- Calories: 250
- Carbohydrates: 12g
- Protein: 28g
- Fat: 10g
- Fiber: 4g
- Sodium: 480mg

Serves

4

Cooking Time

20 minutes

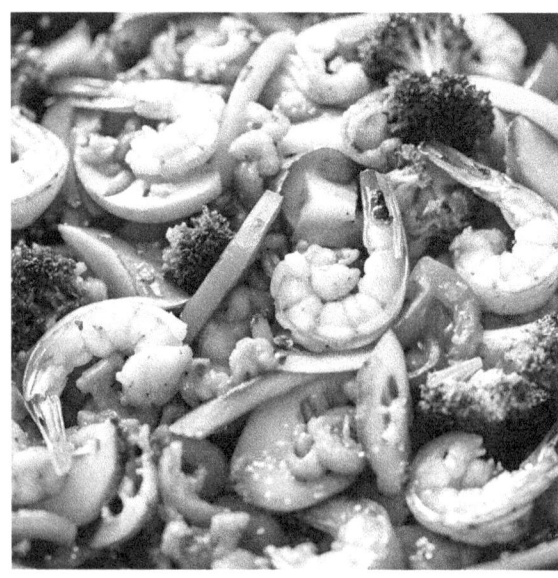

11. Garlic Scallops

Ingredients

- 1 pound sea scallops
- 2 tablespoons olive oil
- 4 garlic cloves, minced
- 1/4 cup fresh lemon juice
- 1/4 cup fresh parsley, chopped
- 1 teaspoon ground black pepper

Instructions

1. Pat the scallops dry with a paper towel.
2. Heat olive oil in a large skillet over medium-high heat.
3. Add scallops to the skillet and cook for 2-3 minutes on each side, until golden brown and cooked through. Remove from the skillet and set aside.
4. In the same skillet, add minced garlic and cook for 1 minute until fragrant.
5. Stir in lemon juice and ground black pepper.
6. Return the scallops to the skillet and cook for another 1-2 minutes, until heated through.
7. Garnish with fresh parsley before serving.
8. Serve hot.

Nutrition Info per Serving

- Calories: 220
- Carbohydrates: 6g
- Protein: 28g
- Fat: 8g
- Fiber: 1g
- Sodium: 340mg

Serves

4

Cooking Time

15 minutes

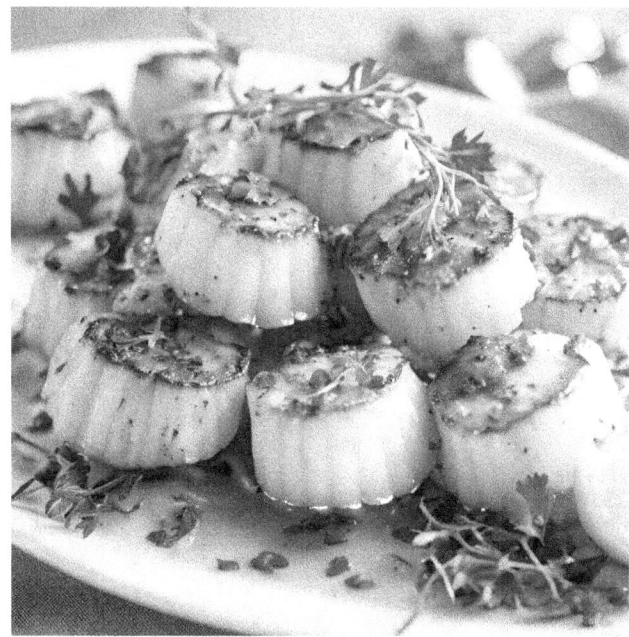

12. Mussels in Tomato Broth

Ingredients

- 2 pounds mussels, cleaned and debearded
- 2 tablespoons olive oil
- 1 onion, chopped
- 3 garlic cloves, minced
- 1 can (14.5 ounces) diced tomatoes (no salt added)
- 1 cup low-sodium vegetable broth
- 1/2 cup white wine (optional, for flavor)
- 1 teaspoon dried thyme
- 1 teaspoon ground black pepper
- 1/4 cup fresh parsley, chopped

Instructions

1. Heat olive oil in a large pot over medium heat. Add onion and garlic, cooking for 3-4 minutes until softened.
2. Stir in diced tomatoes, vegetable broth, white wine (if using), dried thyme, and ground black pepper. Bring to a simmer.
3. Add the mussels to the pot, cover, and cook for 5-7 minutes until the mussels open.
4. Discard any mussels that do not open.
5. Sprinkle with fresh parsley before serving.
6. Serve hot.

Nutrition Info per Serving

- Calories: 240
- Carbohydrates: 10g
- Protein: 28g
- Fat: 8g
- Fiber: 2g
- Sodium: 340mg

Serves

4

Cooking Time

20 minutes

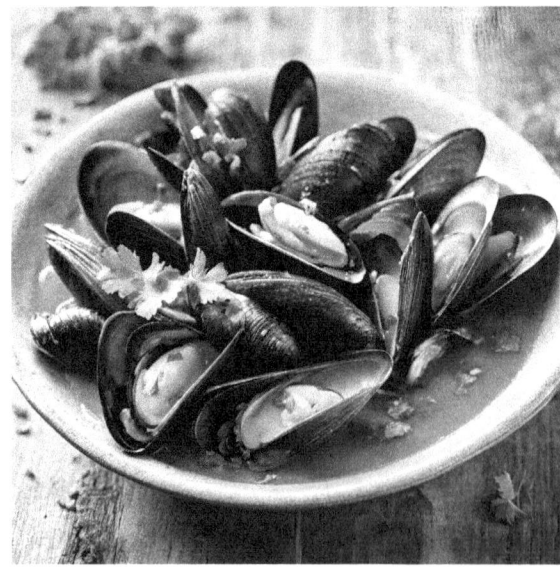

13. Spicy Shrimp Tacos

Ingredients

- 1 pound shrimp, peeled and deveined
- 2 tablespoons olive oil
- 1 teaspoon ground cumin
- 1 teaspoon smoked paprika
- 1/2 teaspoon ground black pepper
- 1/2 teaspoon cayenne pepper
- 8 small whole wheat tortillas
- 1 cup shredded cabbage
- 1/2 cup diced tomatoes
- 1/4 cup red onion, finely chopped
- 1/4 cup fresh cilantro, chopped
- 2 tablespoons fresh lime juice

Instructions

1. In a large bowl, toss the shrimp with olive oil, ground cumin, smoked paprika, ground black pepper, and cayenne pepper until evenly coated.
2. Heat a large skillet over medium-high heat. Add the shrimp and cook for 2-3 minutes on each side until cooked through.
3. Warm the tortillas in a dry skillet or microwave.
4. To assemble the tacos, place shrimp on each tortilla and top with shredded cabbage, diced tomatoes, red onion, and cilantro.
5. Drizzle with fresh lime juice before serving.
6. Serve immediately.

Nutrition Info per Serving

- Calories: 230
- Carbohydrates: 20g
- Protein: 22g
- Fat: 8g
- Fiber: 4g
- Sodium: 400mg

Serves

4 (2 tacos per serving)

Cooking Time

20 minutes

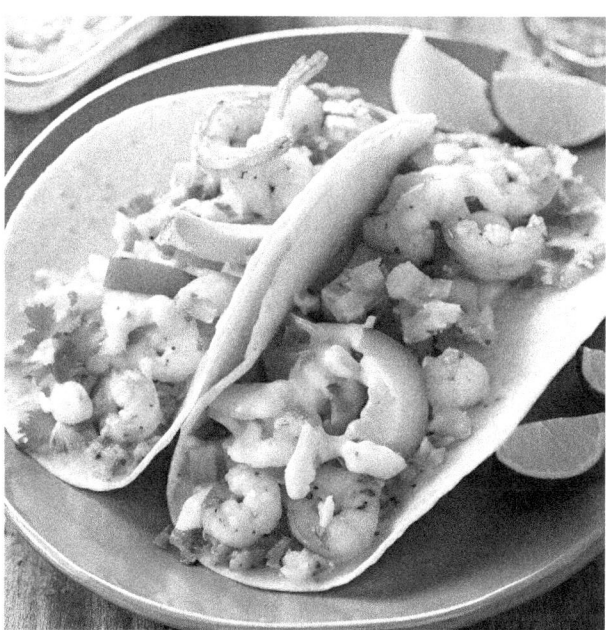

14. Scallop and Pea Risotto

Ingredients

- 1 pound sea scallops
- 1 cup Arborio rice
- 1 tablespoon olive oil
- 1 onion, finely chopped
- 3 garlic cloves, minced
- 4 cups low-sodium vegetable broth, warmed
- 1 cup frozen peas
- 1/4 cup grated Parmesan cheese
- 1/4 cup fresh parsley, chopped
- 1/4 cup fresh lemon juice
- 1 teaspoon ground black pepper

Instructions

1. Heat olive oil in a large skillet over medium heat. Add the onion and garlic, cooking for 3-4 minutes until softened.
2. Add Arborio rice and cook for 2 minutes, stirring constantly.
3. Gradually add the warmed vegetable broth, 1 cup at a time, stirring frequently until the liquid is absorbed before adding more. Continue until the rice is tender and creamy, about 20 minutes.
4. Stir in the peas, Parmesan cheese, and ground black pepper. Cook for an additional 2-3 minutes until the peas are heated through.
5. Meanwhile, in another skillet, sear the scallops over medium-high heat for 2-3 minutes on each side until golden brown and cooked through.
6. Stir lemon juice and fresh parsley into the risotto.
7. Serve the risotto topped with seared scallops.
8. Serve hot.

Nutrition Info per Serving

- Calories: 350
- Carbohydrates: 40g
- Protein: 28g
- Fat: 10g
- Fiber: 4g
- Sodium: 300mg

Serves

4

Cooking Time

30 minutes

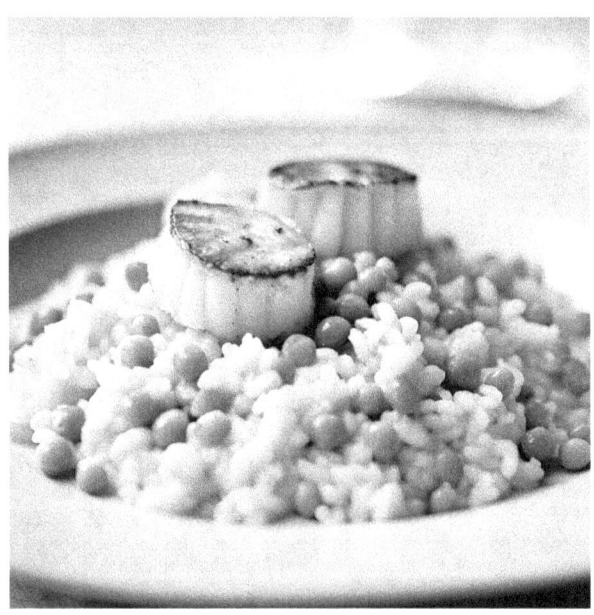

15. Seafood Paella

Ingredients

- 1 pound shrimp, peeled and deveined
- 1 pound mussels, cleaned and debearded
- 1 pound clams, cleaned
- 1 pound squid, cleaned and sliced into rings
- 2 tablespoons olive oil
- 1 onion, chopped
- 3 garlic cloves, minced
- 1 red bell pepper, chopped
- 1 cup Arborio rice
- 1/2 teaspoon ground turmeric
- 1 teaspoon smoked paprika
- 4 cups low-sodium chicken broth
- 1 cup frozen peas
- 1/4 cup fresh parsley, chopped
- 1 lemon, cut into wedges

Instructions

1. Heat olive oil in a large, deep skillet or paella pan over medium heat. Add onion, garlic, and red bell pepper. Cook for 5-7 minutes until vegetables are softened.
2. Stir in the Arborio rice, ground turmeric, and smoked paprika. Cook for 2 minutes, stirring constantly.
3. Add the low-sodium chicken broth and bring to a boil. Reduce heat to low and simmer for 10 minutes.
4. Add shrimp, mussels, clams, and squid to the pan, stirring gently to combine. Cook for another 10-12 minutes, until the seafood is cooked and the rice is tender.
5. Stir in the frozen peas and cook for an additional 2-3 minutes.
6. Sprinkle with fresh parsley and serve with lemon wedges.
7. Serve hot.

Nutrition Info per Serving

- Calories: 360
- Carbohydrates: 40g
- Protein: 32g
- Fat: 10g
- Fiber: 4g
- Sodium: 380mg

Serves
6
Cooking Time
30 minutes

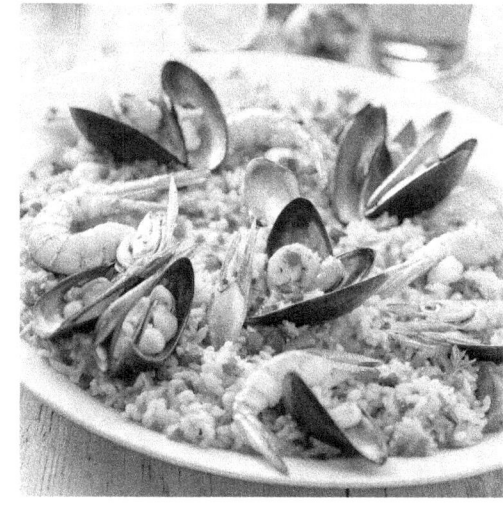

16. Fisherman's Stew

Ingredients

- 1 pound white fish fillets (such as cod or halibut), cut into chunks
- 1 pound shrimp, peeled and deveined
- 1 pound mussels, cleaned and debearded
- 2 tablespoons olive oil
- 1 onion, chopped
- 3 garlic cloves, minced
- 1 fennel bulb, thinly sliced
- 1 can (14.5 ounces) diced tomatoes (no salt added)
- 4 cups low-sodium fish broth
- 1/2 cup dry white wine (optional)
- 1 teaspoon dried thyme
- 1 teaspoon ground black pepper
- 1/4 cup fresh parsley, chopped

Instructions

1. Heat olive oil in a large pot over medium heat. Add onion, garlic, and fennel. Cook for 5-7 minutes until vegetables are softened.
2. Stir in diced tomatoes, fish broth, white wine (if using), dried thyme, and ground black pepper. Bring to a simmer.
3. Add the white fish chunks, shrimp, and mussels to the pot. Cover and cook for 5-7 minutes until the seafood is cooked through and the mussels have opened.
4. Discard any mussels that do not open.
5. Sprinkle with fresh parsley before serving.
6. Serve hot.

Nutrition Info per Serving

- Calories: 320
- Carbohydrates: 10g
- Protein: 36g
- Fat: 12g
- Fiber: 2g
- Sodium: 360mg

Serves
6

Cooking Time
30 minutes

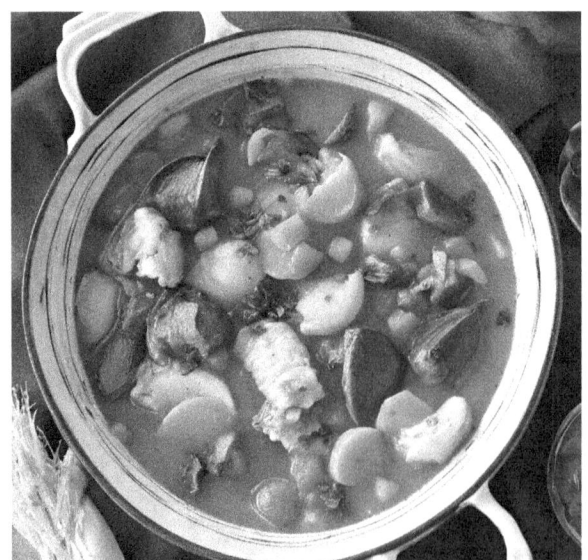

17. Grilled Sea Bass with Mango Salsa

Ingredients

- 4 sea bass fillets (about 6 ounces each)
- 2 tablespoons olive oil
- 1 teaspoon ground black pepper
- 1 mango, diced
- 1/2 red onion, finely chopped
- 1/4 cup fresh cilantro, chopped
- 1 jalapeno, seeded and minced
- 2 tablespoons fresh lime juice

Instructions

1. Preheat the grill to medium-high heat.
2. Brush sea bass fillets with olive oil and sprinkle with ground black pepper.
3. Grill the sea bass for 4-5 minutes on each side, until the fish is cooked through and flakes easily with a fork.
4. In a bowl, combine diced mango, red onion, cilantro, jalapeno, and lime juice. Mix well.
5. Serve the grilled sea bass topped with mango salsa.
6. Serve hot.

Nutrition Info per Serving

- Calories: 280
- Carbohydrates: 10g
- Protein: 32g
- Fat: 14g
- Fiber: 2g
- Sodium: 140mg

Serves

4

Cooking Time

15 minutes

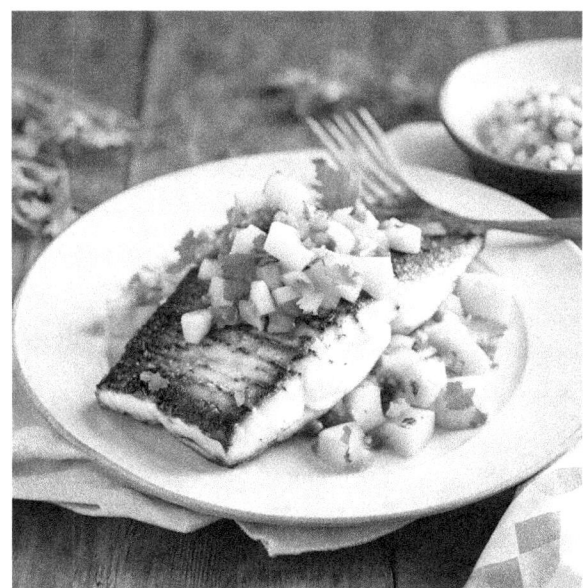

18. Baked Trout with Walnut Crust

Ingredients

- 4 trout fillets (about 6 ounces each)
- 1/2 cup walnuts, finely chopped
- 1/4 cup whole wheat breadcrumbs
- 2 tablespoons olive oil
- 1 tablespoon fresh parsley, chopped
- 1 teaspoon ground black pepper
- 1 lemon, sliced

Instructions

1. Preheat the oven to 375°F (190°C).
2. In a small bowl, combine chopped walnuts, whole wheat breadcrumbs, olive oil, fresh parsley, and ground black pepper.
3. Place trout fillets on a baking sheet lined with parchment paper. Press the walnut mixture onto the top of each fillet.
4. Bake for 15-20 minutes, until the fish is cooked through and the crust is golden brown.
5. Serve with lemon slices.
6. Serve hot.

Nutrition Info per Serving

- Calories: 340
- Carbohydrates: 6g
- Protein: 34g
- Fat: 20g
- Fiber: 2g
- Sodium: 120mg

Serves

4

Cooking Time

20 minutes

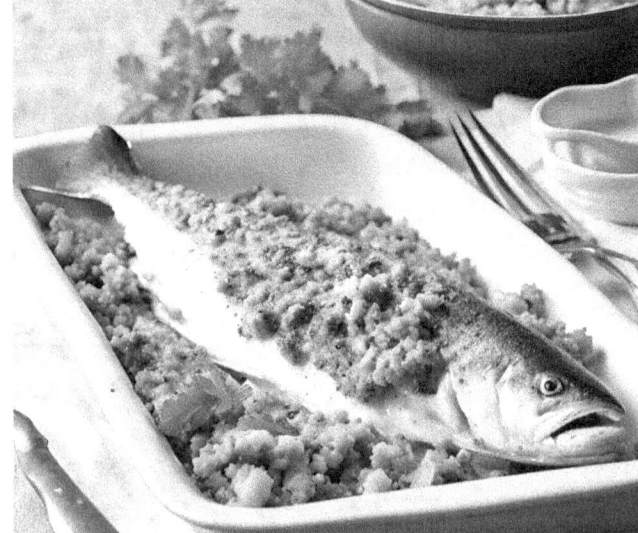

19. Cod with Greek Salad

Ingredients

- 4 cod fillets (about 6 ounces each)
- 2 tablespoons olive oil
- 1 teaspoon dried oregano
- 1 teaspoon ground black pepper
- 2 cups cherry tomatoes, halved
- 1 cucumber, diced
- 1/4 red onion, thinly sliced
- 1/4 cup Kalamata olives, pitted and sliced
- 1/4 cup feta cheese, crumbled
- 2 tablespoons fresh lemon juice
- 1 tablespoon red wine vinegar

Instructions

1. Preheat the oven to 375°F (190°C).
2. Place cod fillets on a baking sheet lined with parchment paper. Drizzle with olive oil and sprinkle with dried oregano and ground black pepper.
3. Bake for 15-20 minutes, until the fish is cooked through and flakes easily with a fork.
4. In a large bowl, combine cherry tomatoes, cucumber, red onion, olives, and feta cheese.
5. In a small bowl, whisk together lemon juice and red wine vinegar. Pour over the salad and toss to combine.
6. Serve the baked cod with the Greek salad on the side.
7. Serve hot.

Nutrition Info per Serving

- Calories: 290
- Carbohydrates: 10g
- Protein: 34g
- Fat: 14g
- Fiber: 3g
- Sodium: 270mg

Serves

4

Cooking Time

20 minutes

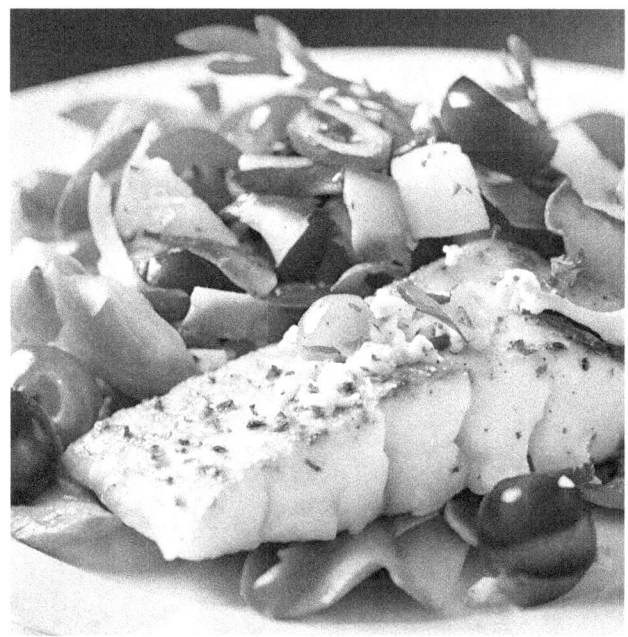

20. Sushi Rolls with Brown Rice

Ingredients

- 2 cups cooked brown rice, cooled
- 2 tablespoons rice vinegar
- 1 tablespoon honey
- 4 nori sheets
- 1 cucumber, julienned
- 1 avocado, sliced
- 1 carrot, julienned
- 1/2 pound cooked shrimp, sliced lengthwise
- 2 tablespoons low-sodium soy sauce
- 1 teaspoon ground black pepper

Instructions

1. In a small bowl, mix the rice vinegar and honey. Stir into the cooled brown rice.
2. Place a nori sheet on a bamboo sushi mat. Spread a thin layer of brown rice over the nori, leaving a 1-inch border at the top.
3. Arrange cucumber, avocado, carrot, and shrimp in a line along the bottom edge of the nori sheet.
4. Roll the sushi tightly using the bamboo mat, sealing the edge with a little water.
5. Repeat with remaining ingredients.
6. Slice each roll into 8 pieces.
7. Serve with low-sodium soy sauce and a sprinkle of ground black pepper.
8. Serve immediately.

Nutrition Info per Serving

- Calories: 250
- Carbohydrates: 32g
- Protein: 16g
- Fat: 8g
- Fiber: 5g
- Sodium: 300mg

Serves
4
Cooking Time
30 minutes

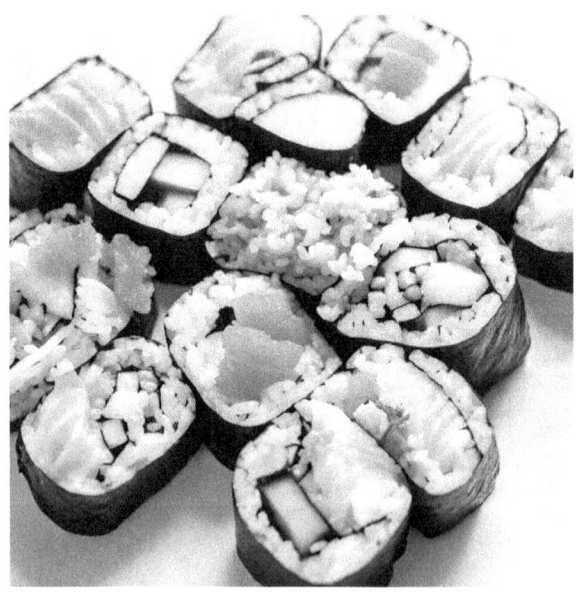

21. Kedgeree with Smoked Fish

Ingredients

- 1 pound smoked haddock fillets
- 1 cup basmati rice
- 3 cups low-sodium chicken broth
- 2 tablespoons olive oil
- 1 onion, finely chopped
- 2 garlic cloves, minced
- 1 tablespoon curry powder
- 1/2 cup frozen peas
- 3 hard-boiled eggs, chopped
- 1/4 cup fresh parsley, chopped
- 1 lemon, cut into wedges

Instructions

1. In a large pot, bring the low-sodium chicken broth to a simmer. Add the smoked haddock fillets and poach for 8-10 minutes until cooked through. Remove the fish and set aside, reserving the broth.
2. In a large skillet, heat olive oil over medium heat. Add the onion and garlic, cooking for 3-4 minutes until softened.
3. Stir in the curry powder and cook for 1 minute.
4. Add the basmati rice and reserved broth to the skillet. Bring to a boil, then reduce heat, cover, and simmer for 15-20 minutes until the rice is tender.
5. Stir in the frozen peas and chopped hard-boiled eggs. Cook for an additional 2-3 minutes.
6. Flake the poached haddock into the skillet and gently stir to combine.
7. Sprinkle with fresh parsley and serve with lemon wedges.
8. Serve hot.

Nutrition Info per Serving

- Calories: 350
- Carbohydrates: 40g
- Protein: 28g
- Fat: 12g
- Fiber: 4g
- Sodium: 300mg

Serves

4

Cooking Time

30 minutes

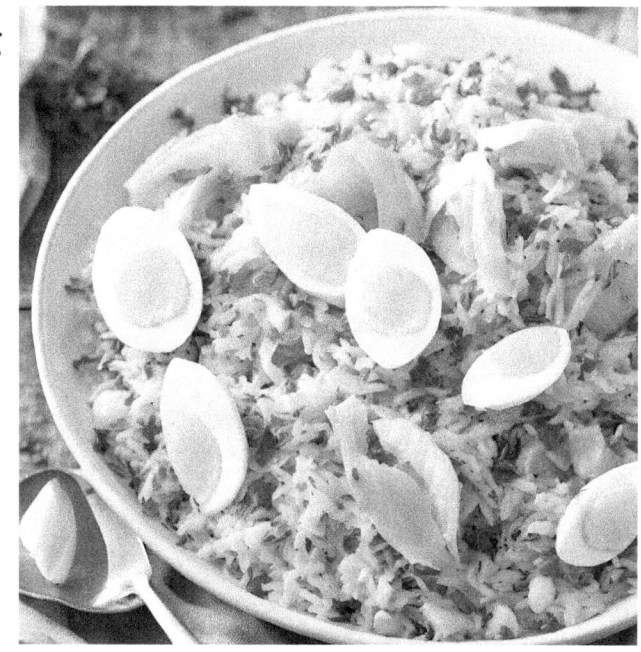

22. Fish Fillet with Citrus Quinoa

Ingredients

- 4 fish fillets (such as cod or tilapia, about 6 ounces each)
- 2 tablespoons olive oil
- 1 teaspoon ground black pepper
- 1 cup quinoa
- 2 cups low-sodium vegetable broth
- 1 orange, juiced and zested
- 1 lemon, juiced and zested
- 1/4 cup fresh parsley, chopped

Instructions

1. Preheat oven to 375°F (190°C).
2. Brush the fish fillets with 1 tablespoon of olive oil and sprinkle with ground black pepper. Place on a baking sheet lined with parchment paper.
3. Bake for 15-20 minutes, until the fish is cooked through and flakes easily with a fork.
4. Meanwhile, in a medium pot, bring the vegetable broth to a boil. Add the quinoa, reduce heat, cover, and simmer for 15 minutes until the liquid is absorbed and the quinoa is tender.
5. In a small bowl, combine the orange juice, lemon juice, orange zest, lemon zest, and remaining olive oil.
6. Fluff the cooked quinoa with a fork and stir in the citrus mixture and chopped parsley.
7. Serve the fish fillets on a bed of citrus quinoa.
8. Serve hot.

Nutrition Info per Serving

- Calories: 320
- Carbohydrates: 30g
- Protein: 34g
- Fat: 10g
- Fiber: 5g
- Sodium: 180mg

Serves

4

Cooking Time

25 minutes

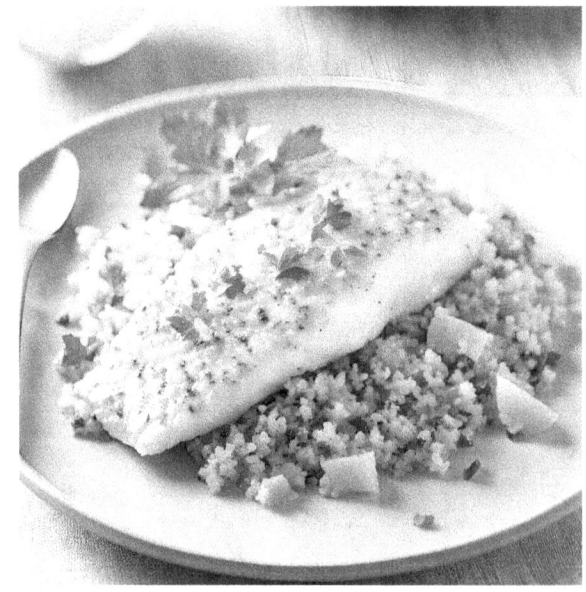

23. Spicy Tuna Poke Bowl

Ingredients

- 1 pound sushi-grade tuna, diced
- 2 tablespoons low-sodium soy sauce
- 1 tablespoon sesame oil
- 1 tablespoon sriracha
- 1 teaspoon grated ginger
- 2 cups cooked brown rice, cooled
- 1 avocado, sliced
- 1 cucumber, julienned
- 1 carrot, julienned
- 2 green onions, sliced
- 1 tablespoon sesame seeds

Instructions

1. In a medium bowl, combine diced tuna, soy sauce, sesame oil, sriracha, and grated ginger. Mix well and let marinate for 10 minutes.
2. Divide the cooked brown rice into four bowls.
3. Top each bowl with marinated tuna, avocado slices, cucumber, carrot, and green onions.
4. Sprinkle with sesame seeds.
5. Serve immediately.

Nutrition Info per Serving

- Calories: 400
- Carbohydrates: 35g
- Protein: 34g
- Fat: 14g
- Fiber: 6g
- Sodium: 420mg

Serves

4

Cooking Time

20 minutes

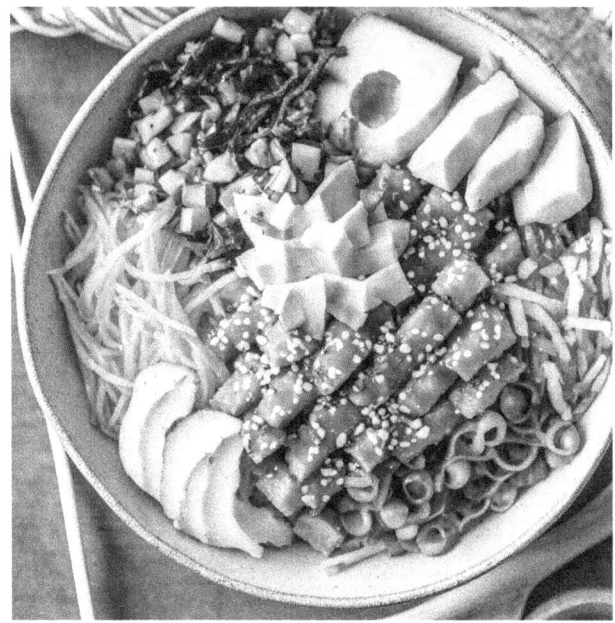

24. Seafood and Spinach Lasagna

Ingredients

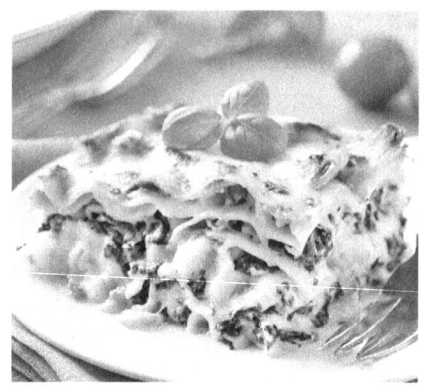

- 1 pound shrimp, peeled and deveined
- 1 pound scallops
- 2 tablespoons olive oil
- 1 onion, chopped
- 3 garlic cloves, minced
- 4 cups fresh spinach, chopped
- 1 can (14.5 ounces) diced tomatoes (no salt added)
- 1 teaspoon dried oregano
- 1 teaspoon ground black pepper
- 9 whole wheat lasagna noodles, cooked
- 2 cups ricotta cheese
- 1 cup shredded mozzarella cheese
- 1/4 cup grated Parmesan cheese

Instructions

1. Preheat oven to 375°F (190°C).
2. In a large skillet, heat olive oil over medium heat. Add onion and garlic, cooking for 3-4 minutes until softened.
3. Stir in the shrimp and scallops, cooking for 5-7 minutes until the seafood is cooked through. Remove from the skillet and set aside.
4. In the same skillet, add chopped spinach, diced tomatoes, dried oregano, and ground black pepper. Cook for 5 minutes until the spinach is wilted and the sauce thickens.
5. In a 9x13-inch baking dish, spread a thin layer of the spinach and tomato sauce.
6. Arrange 3 lasagna noodles on top, followed by half of the seafood mixture, half of the ricotta cheese, and half of the remaining sauce.
7. Repeat the layers, ending with the final 3 lasagna noodles and the remaining sauce.
8. Sprinkle with shredded mozzarella and grated Parmesan cheese.
9. Cover with foil and bake for 25 minutes. Remove the foil and bake for an additional 10 minutes until the cheese is melted and bubbly.
10. Let cool for 10 minutes before serving.
11. Serve hot.

Nutrition Info per Serving

- Calories: 380   Carbohydrates: 30g   Protein: **36g**   Fat: 14g
- Fiber: 5g
- Sodium: 320mg

Serves

6

Cooking Time

45 minutes

25. Lemon Butter Scampi

Ingredients

- 1 pound shrimp, peeled and deveined
- 3 tablespoons olive oil
- 4 garlic cloves, minced
- 1/4 cup fresh lemon juice
- 1/4 cup low-sodium chicken broth
- 2 tablespoons unsalted butter
- 1/4 cup fresh parsley, chopped
- 1 teaspoon ground black pepper
- 1 lemon, sliced for garnish

Instructions

1. Heat olive oil in a large skillet over medium heat. Add minced garlic and cook for 1-2 minutes until fragrant.
2. Add the shrimp and cook for 2-3 minutes on each side until pink and cooked through. Remove from the skillet and set aside.
3. In the same skillet, add lemon juice and chicken broth. Bring to a simmer.
4. Stir in unsalted butter until melted.
5. Return the shrimp to the skillet and cook for an additional 2 minutes until heated through.
6. Sprinkle with fresh parsley and ground black pepper.
7. Serve garnished with lemon slices.
8. Serve hot.

Nutrition Info per Serving

- Calories: 280
- Carbohydrates: 4g
- Protein: 28g
- Fat: 18g
- Fiber: 1g
- Sodium: 260mg

Serves

4

Cooking Time

15 minutes

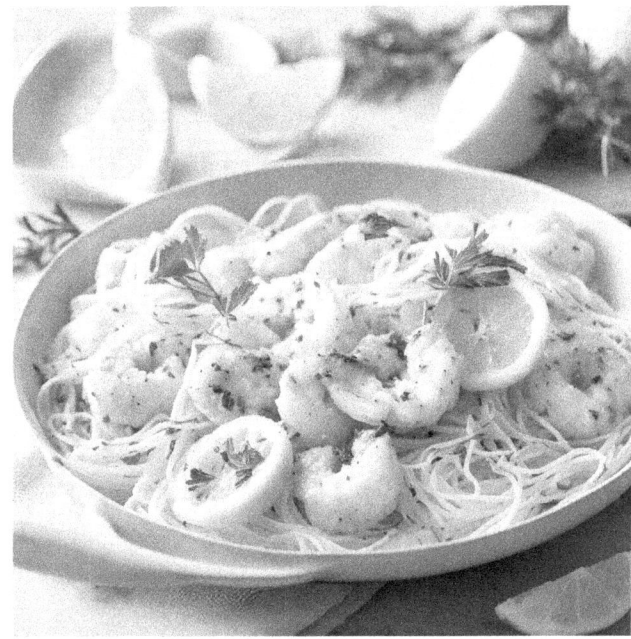

26. Baked Catfish with Sweet Potato Fries
Ingredients
- 4 catfish fillets (about 6 ounces each)
- 2 tablespoons olive oil
- 1 teaspoon ground paprika
- 1 teaspoon ground black pepper
- 4 large sweet potatoes, cut into fries
- 2 tablespoons olive oil
- 1 teaspoon garlic powder

Instructions
1. Preheat oven to 400°F (200°C).
2. Place the catfish fillets on a baking sheet lined with parchment paper. Brush with olive oil and sprinkle with ground paprika and ground black pepper.
3. In a large bowl, toss the sweet potato fries with olive oil and garlic powder.
4. Spread the sweet potato fries on another baking sheet lined with parchment paper.
5. Bake the catfish and sweet potato fries for 25-30 minutes, until the fish is cooked through and flakes easily with a fork and the fries are crispy.
6. Serve the baked catfish with the sweet potato fries.
7. Serve hot.

Nutrition Info per Serving
- Calories: 350
- Carbohydrates: 45g
- Protein: 28g
- Fat: 12g
- Fiber: 8g
- Sodium: 200mg

Serves
4
Cooking Time
30 minutes

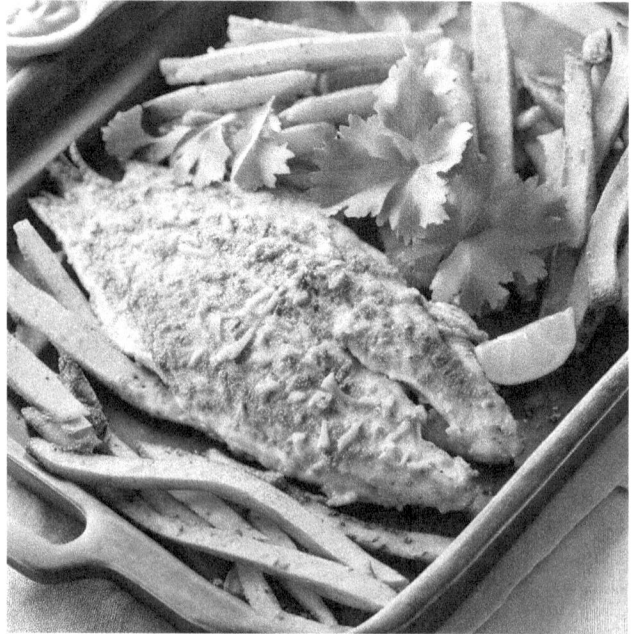

Soup & Stew Recipes

1. Japanese Miso-Glazed Cod
Ingredients
- 4 cod fillets (about 6 ounces each)
- 1/4 cup white miso paste
- 2 tablespoons rice vinegar
- 2 tablespoons mirin
- 1 tablespoon honey
- 1 tablespoon low-sodium soy sauce
- 1 tablespoon fresh ginger, grated
- 2 green onions, sliced

Instructions
1. Preheat the oven to 400°F (200°C).
2. In a small bowl, whisk together miso paste, rice vinegar, mirin, honey, soy sauce, and grated ginger until smooth.
3. Place cod fillets on a baking sheet lined with parchment paper.
4. Brush the miso glaze evenly over each fillet.
5. Bake for 12-15 minutes, until the fish is cooked through and flakes easily with a fork.
6. Garnish with sliced green onions before serving.
7. Serve hot.

Nutrition Info per Serving
- Calories: 260
- Carbohydrates: 12g
- Protein: 28g
- Fat: 10g
- Fiber: 1g
- Sodium: 300mg

Serves
4
Cooking Time
15 minutes

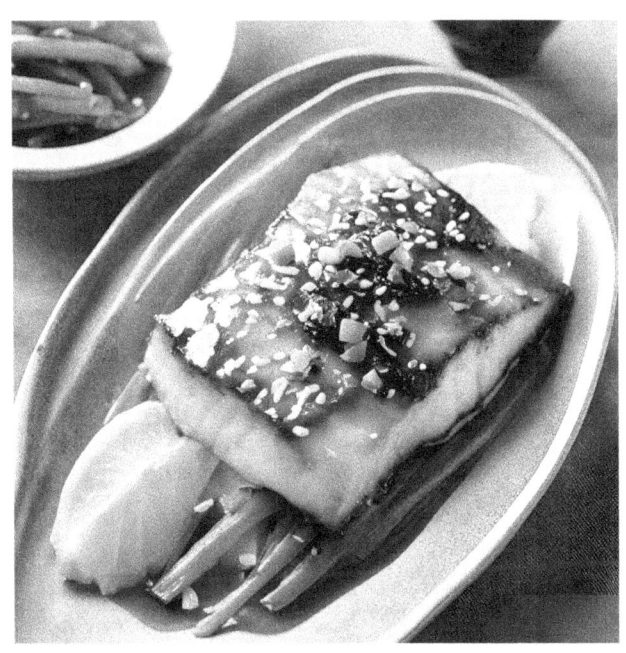

2. Carrot Ginger Soup

Ingredients

- 2 tablespoons olive oil
- 1 onion, chopped
- 4 cups carrots, peeled and chopped
- 2 garlic cloves, minced
- 2 tablespoons fresh ginger, grated
- 4 cups low-sodium vegetable broth
- 1 cup unsweetened almond milk
- 1 teaspoon ground cumin
- 1/2 teaspoon ground black pepper
- 1/4 cup fresh parsley, chopped (optional, for garnish)

Instructions

1. Heat olive oil in a large pot over medium heat. Add onion and garlic, cooking for 3-4 minutes until softened.
2. Add chopped carrots and grated ginger. Cook for another 5 minutes, stirring occasionally.
3. Stir in vegetable broth, ground cumin, and ground black pepper. Bring to a boil, then reduce heat and simmer for 20-25 minutes until carrots are tender.
4. Remove from heat and use an immersion blender to puree the soup until smooth.
5. Stir in unsweetened almond milk and return to heat for another 5 minutes until heated through.
6. Garnish with fresh parsley before serving, if desired.
7. Serve hot.

Nutrition Info per Serving

- Calories: 180
- Carbohydrates: 24g
- Protein: 3g
- Fat: 8g
- Fiber: 6g
- Sodium: 200mg

Serves
4

Cooking Time
30 minutes

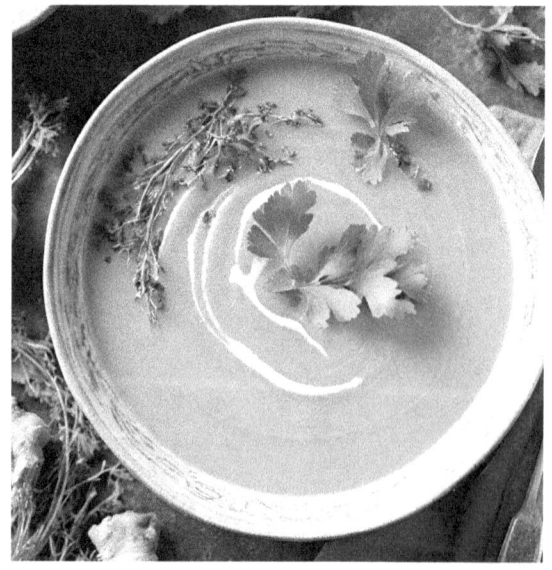

3. Roasted Butternut Squash Soup

Ingredients

- 2 pounds butternut squash, peeled and cubed
- 2 tablespoons olive oil
- 1 onion, chopped
- 3 garlic cloves, minced
- 4 cups low-sodium vegetable broth
- 1 teaspoon ground cinnamon
- 1/2 teaspoon ground nutmeg
- 1/2 teaspoon ground black pepper
- 1 cup unsweetened coconut milk
- 1/4 cup fresh cilantro, chopped (optional, for garnish)

Instructions

1. Preheat the oven to 400°F (200°C).
2. Toss butternut squash cubes with 1 tablespoon of olive oil and spread on a baking sheet. Roast for 25-30 minutes until tender and lightly browned.
3. In a large pot, heat the remaining olive oil over medium heat. Add chopped onion and minced garlic, cooking for 3-4 minutes until softened.
4. Add roasted butternut squash, vegetable broth, ground cinnamon, ground nutmeg, and ground black pepper to the pot. Bring to a boil, then reduce heat and simmer for 15-20 minutes.
5. Remove from heat and use an immersion blender to puree the soup until smooth.
6. Stir in unsweetened coconut milk and return to heat for another 5 minutes until heated through.
7. Garnish with fresh cilantro before serving, if desired.
8. Serve hot.

Nutrition Info per Serving

- Calories: 220
- Carbohydrates: 30g
- Protein: 3g
- Fat: 12g
- Fiber: 6g
- Sodium: 180mg

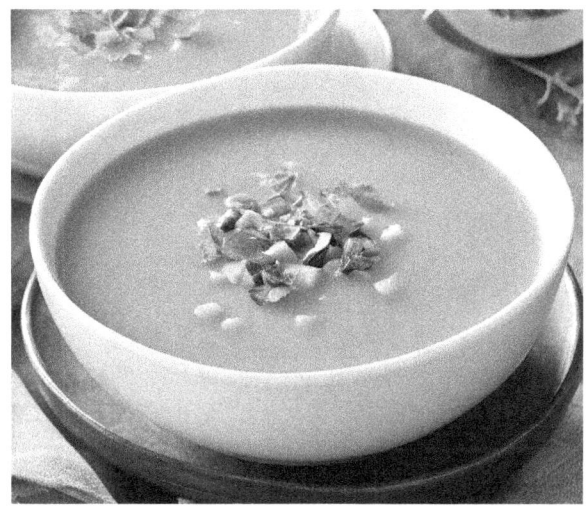

Serves
4
Cooking Time
45 minutes

4. Broccoli and Almond Soup

Ingredients

- 2 tablespoons olive oil
- 1 onion, chopped
- 4 cups broccoli florets
- 2 garlic cloves, minced
- 1/4 cup slivered almonds, toasted
- 4 cups low-sodium vegetable broth
- 1 cup unsweetened almond milk
- 1 teaspoon ground black pepper
- 1/4 cup fresh basil, chopped (optional, for garnish)

Instructions

1. Heat olive oil in a large pot over medium heat. Add chopped onion and minced garlic, cooking for 3-4 minutes until softened.
2. Add broccoli florets and toasted almonds. Cook for another 5 minutes, stirring occasionally.
3. Stir in vegetable broth and ground black pepper. Bring to a boil, then reduce heat and simmer for 15-20 minutes until broccoli is tender.
4. Remove from heat and use an immersion blender to puree the soup until smooth.
5. Stir in unsweetened almond milk and return to heat for another 5 minutes until heated through.
6. Garnish with fresh basil before serving, if desired.
7. Serve hot.

Nutrition Info per Serving

- Calories: 190
- Carbohydrates: 12g
- Protein: 6g
- Fat: 14g
- Fiber: 4g
- Sodium: 160mg

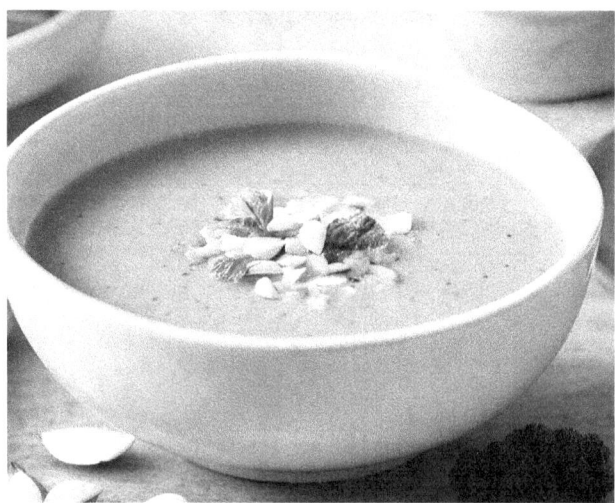

Serves

4

Cooking Time

30 minutes

5. Spicy Sweet Potato Soup

Ingredients

- 2 tablespoons olive oil
- 1 onion, chopped
- 3 garlic cloves, minced
- 2 pounds sweet potatoes, peeled and cubed
- 4 cups low-sodium vegetable broth
- 1 teaspoon ground cumin
- 1 teaspoon smoked paprika
- 1/2 teaspoon ground black pepper
- 1/4 teaspoon cayenne pepper
- 1 cup unsweetened coconut milk
- 1/4 cup fresh cilantro, chopped (optional, for garnish)

Instructions

1. Heat olive oil in a large pot over medium heat. Add chopped onion and minced garlic, cooking for 3-4 minutes until softened.
2. Add cubed sweet potatoes, vegetable broth, ground cumin, smoked paprika, ground black pepper, and cayenne pepper. Bring to a boil, then reduce heat and simmer for 20-25 minutes until sweet potatoes are tender.
3. Remove from heat and use an immersion blender to puree the soup until smooth.
4. Stir in unsweetened coconut milk and return to heat for another 5 minutes until heated through.
5. Garnish with fresh cilantro before serving, if desired.
6. Serve hot.

Nutrition Info per Serving

- Calories: 250
- Carbohydrates: 34g
- Protein: 3g
- Fat: 12g
- Fiber: 6g
- Sodium: 200mg

Serves

4

Cooking Time

30 minutes

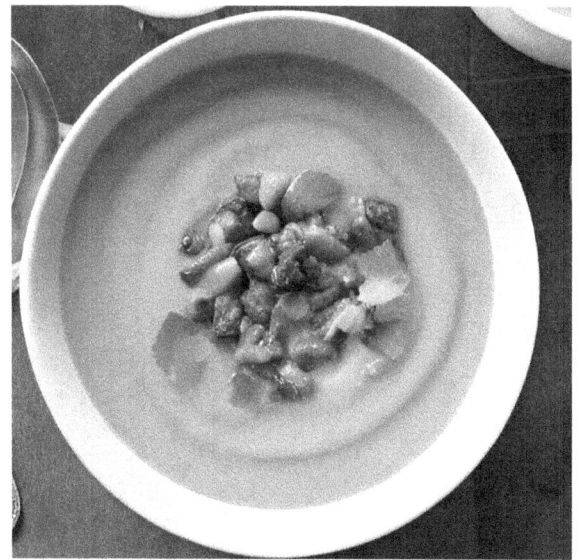

6. Cabbage Detox Soup

Ingredients

- 2 tablespoons olive oil
- 1 onion, chopped
- 3 garlic cloves, minced
- 4 cups cabbage, chopped
- 2 carrots, sliced
- 2 celery stalks, sliced
- 1 zucchini, diced
- 1 can (14.5 ounces) diced tomatoes (no salt added)
- 4 cups low-sodium vegetable broth
- 1 teaspoon dried thyme
- 1 teaspoon ground black pepper
- 1/4 cup fresh parsley, chopped (optional, for garnish)

Instructions

1. Heat olive oil in a large pot over medium heat. Add onion and garlic, cooking for 3-4 minutes until softened.
2. Add chopped cabbage, carrots, celery, and zucchini. Cook for another 5 minutes, stirring occasionally.
3. Stir in diced tomatoes, vegetable broth, dried thyme, and ground black pepper. Bring to a boil, then reduce heat and simmer for 20-25 minutes until vegetables are tender.
4. Garnish with fresh parsley before serving, if desired.
5. Serve hot.

Nutrition Info per Serving

- Calories: 120
- Carbohydrates: 20g
- Protein: 3g
- Fat: 5g
- Fiber: 6g
- Sodium: 180mg

Serves

4

Cooking Time

30 minutes

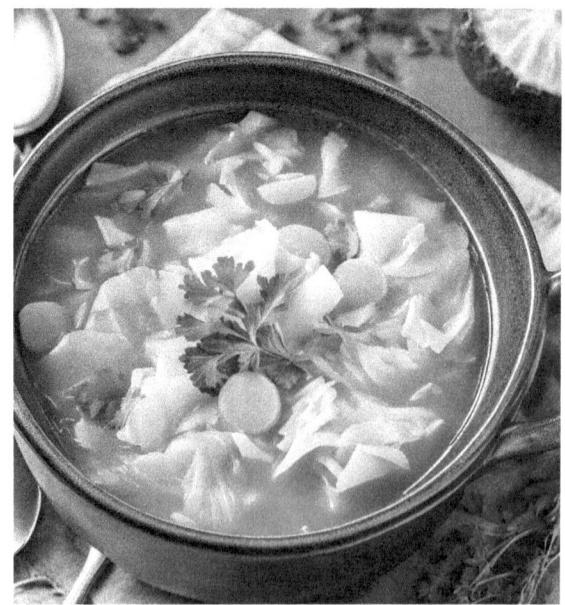

7. Cream of Mushroom Soup

Ingredients

- 2 tablespoons olive oil
- 1 onion, chopped
- 3 garlic cloves, minced
- 1 pound mushrooms, sliced
- 4 cups low-sodium vegetable broth
- 1 teaspoon dried thyme
- 1 teaspoon ground black pepper
- 1 cup unsweetened almond milk
- 1/4 cup fresh parsley, chopped (optional, for garnish)

Instructions

1. Heat olive oil in a large pot over medium heat. Add onion and garlic, cooking for 3-4 minutes until softened.
2. Add sliced mushrooms and cook for another 5-7 minutes until mushrooms are browned and tender.
3. Stir in vegetable broth, dried thyme, and ground black pepper. Bring to a boil, then reduce heat and simmer for 15-20 minutes.
4. Remove from heat and use an immersion blender to puree the soup until smooth.
5. Stir in unsweetened almond milk and return to heat for another 5 minutes until heated through.
6. Garnish with fresh parsley before serving, if desired.
7. Serve hot.

Nutrition Info per Serving

- Calories: 150
- Carbohydrates: 14g
- Protein: 4g
- Fat: 8g
- Fiber: 3g
- Sodium: 160mg

Serves

4

Cooking Time

30 minutes

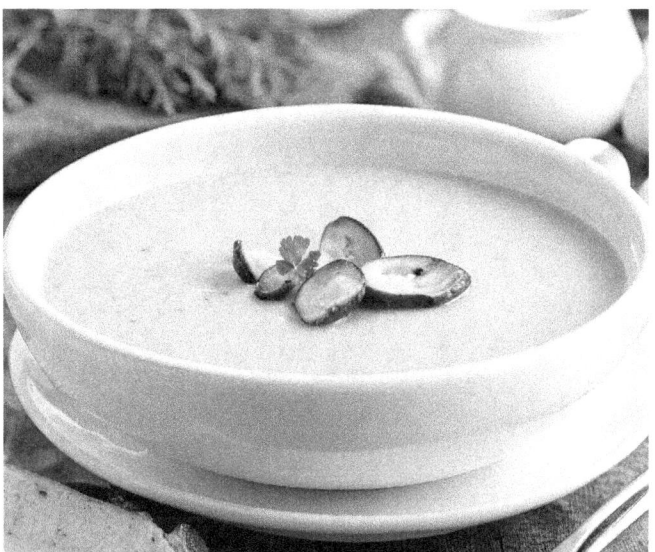

8. Beetroot and Ginger Soup

Ingredients

- 2 tablespoons olive oil
- 1 onion, chopped
- 3 garlic cloves, minced
- 4 medium beets, peeled and diced
- 2 carrots, sliced
- 1 tablespoon fresh ginger, grated
- 4 cups low-sodium vegetable broth
- 1 teaspoon ground cumin
- 1 teaspoon ground black pepper
- 1/4 cup fresh dill, chopped (optional, for garnish)

Instructions

1. Heat olive oil in a large pot over medium heat. Add onion and garlic, cooking for 3-4 minutes until softened.
2. Add diced beets, carrots, and grated ginger. Cook for another 5 minutes, stirring occasionally.
3. Stir in vegetable broth, ground cumin, and ground black pepper. Bring to a boil, then reduce heat and simmer for 25-30 minutes until beets and carrots are tender.
4. Remove from heat and use an immersion blender to puree the soup until smooth.
5. Garnish with fresh dill before serving, if desired.
6. Serve hot.

Nutrition Info per Serving

- Calories: 180
- Carbohydrates: 28g
- Protein: 4g
- Fat: 8g
- Fiber: 6g
- Sodium: 170mg

Serves

4

Cooking Time

40 minutes

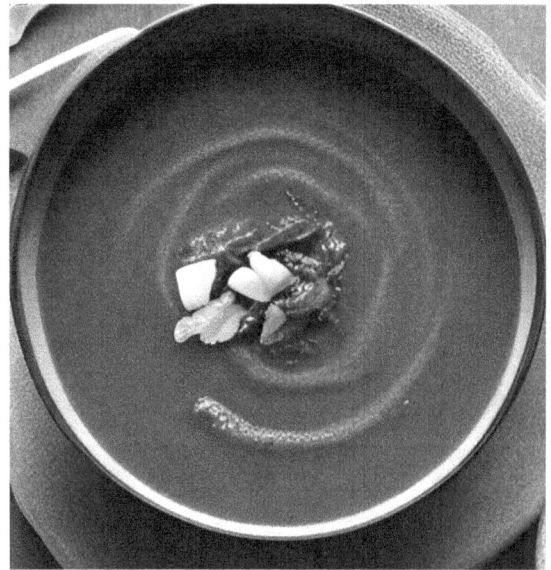

9. Chicken Noodle Soup

Ingredients

- 1 tablespoon olive oil
- 1 onion, chopped
- 3 garlic cloves, minced
- 2 carrots, sliced
- 2 celery stalks, sliced
- 8 cups low-sodium chicken broth
- 2 cups cooked chicken breast, shredded
- 1 cup whole wheat egg noodles
- 1 teaspoon dried thyme
- 1 teaspoon ground black pepper
- 1/4 cup fresh parsley, chopped (optional, for garnish)

Instructions

1. Heat olive oil in a large pot over medium heat. Add onion and garlic, cooking for 3-4 minutes until softened.
2. Add sliced carrots and celery. Cook for another 5 minutes, stirring occasionally.
3. Stir in chicken broth, shredded chicken, whole wheat egg noodles, dried thyme, and ground black pepper. Bring to a boil, then reduce heat and simmer for 10-15 minutes until the noodles are tender.
4. Garnish with fresh parsley before serving, if desired.
5. Serve hot.

Nutrition Info per Serving

- Calories: 250
- Carbohydrates: 20g
- Protein: 25g
- Fat: 8g
- Fiber: 3g
- Sodium: 200mg

Serves

6

Cooking Time

30 minutes

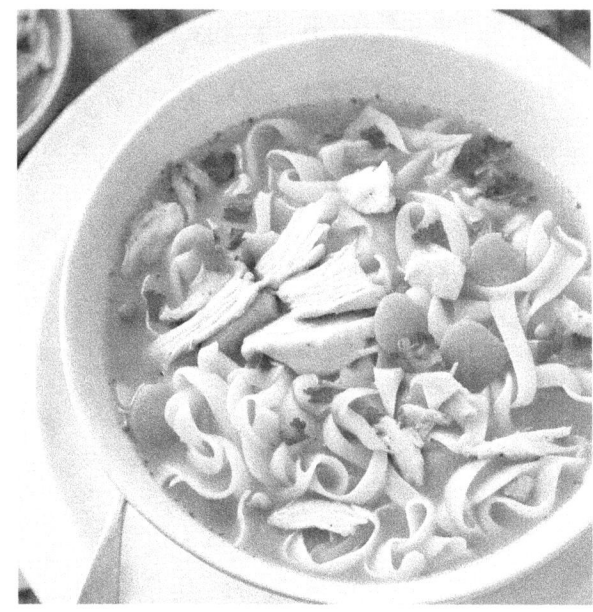

10. Turkey and White Bean Chili

Ingredients

- 1 pound ground turkey
- 2 tablespoons olive oil
- 1 onion, chopped
- 3 garlic cloves, minced
- 1 red bell pepper, chopped
- 1 green bell pepper, chopped
- 1 can (14.5 ounces) diced tomatoes (no salt added)
- 2 cups low-sodium chicken broth
- 1 can (15 ounces) white beans, drained and rinsed
- 1 tablespoon chili powder
- 1 teaspoon ground cumin
- 1 teaspoon ground black pepper
- 1/4 cup fresh cilantro, chopped (optional, for garnish)

Instructions

1. Heat olive oil in a large pot over medium heat. Add ground turkey and cook until browned, about 5-7 minutes.
2. Add onion and garlic, cooking for 3-4 minutes until softened.
3. Stir in red and green bell peppers, cooking for another 5 minutes.
4. Add diced tomatoes, chicken broth, white beans, chili powder, ground cumin, and ground black pepper. Bring to a boil, then reduce heat and simmer for 20-25 minutes.
5. Garnish with fresh cilantro before serving, if desired.
6. Serve hot.

Nutrition Info per Serving

- Calories: 280
- Carbohydrates: 24g
- Protein: 28g
- Fat: 10g
- Fiber: 6g
- Sodium: 240mg

Serves

4

Cooking Time

30 minutes

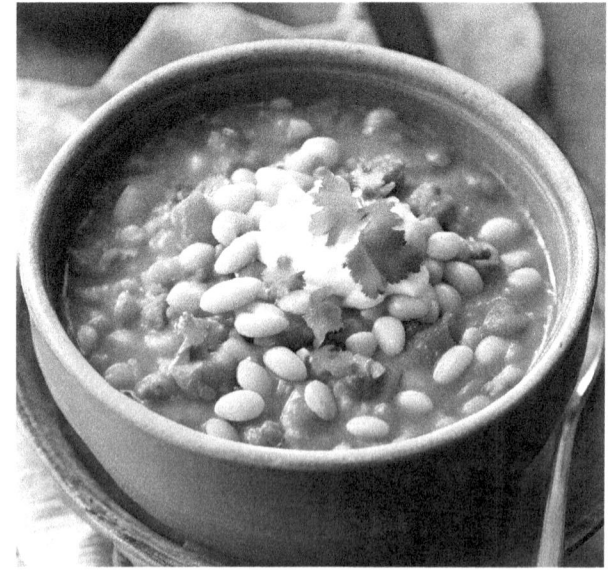

11. Lentil and Spinach Soup

Ingredients

- 2 tablespoons olive oil
- 1 onion, chopped
- 3 garlic cloves, minced
- 2 carrots, diced
- 2 celery stalks, diced
- 1 cup dried lentils, rinsed
- 4 cups low-sodium vegetable broth
- 2 cups water
- 1 teaspoon ground cumin
- 1 teaspoon ground black pepper
- 4 cups fresh spinach, chopped
- 1/4 cup fresh parsley, chopped (optional, for garnish)

Instructions

1. Heat olive oil in a large pot over medium heat. Add onion and garlic, cooking for 3-4 minutes until softened.
2. Add carrots and celery, cooking for another 5 minutes.
3. Stir in lentils, vegetable broth, water, ground cumin, and ground black pepper. Bring to a boil, then reduce heat and simmer for 25-30 minutes until lentils are tender.
4. Stir in chopped spinach and cook for an additional 5 minutes until wilted.
5. Garnish with fresh parsley before serving, if desired.
6. Serve hot.

Nutrition Info per Serving

- Calories: 230
- Carbohydrates: 32g
- Protein: 10g
- Fat: 8g
- Fiber: 10g
- Sodium: 180mg

Serves

4

Cooking Time

35 minutes

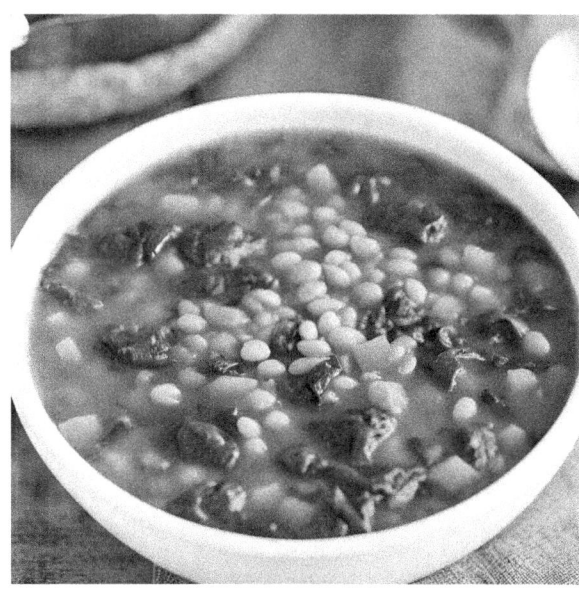

12. Pea and Ham Soup

Ingredients

- 2 tablespoons olive oil
- 1 onion, chopped
- 3 garlic cloves, minced
- 2 cups split peas, rinsed
- 1 ham hock
- 4 cups low-sodium vegetable broth
- 4 cups water
- 2 carrots, diced
- 2 celery stalks, diced
- 1 teaspoon dried thyme
- 1 teaspoon ground black pepper
- 1/4 cup fresh dill, chopped (optional, for garnish)

Instructions

1. Heat olive oil in a large pot over medium heat. Add onion and garlic, cooking for 3-4 minutes until softened.
2. Add split peas, ham hock, vegetable broth, water, carrots, celery, dried thyme, and ground black pepper. Bring to a boil, then reduce heat and simmer for 1.5 to 2 hours until peas are tender and the soup has thickened.
3. Remove the ham hock, shred the meat, and return it to the pot.
4. Garnish with fresh dill before serving, if desired.
5. Serve hot.

Nutrition Info per Serving

- Calories: 300
- Carbohydrates: 40g
- Protein: 18g
- Fat: 10g
- Fiber: 12g
- Sodium: 300mg

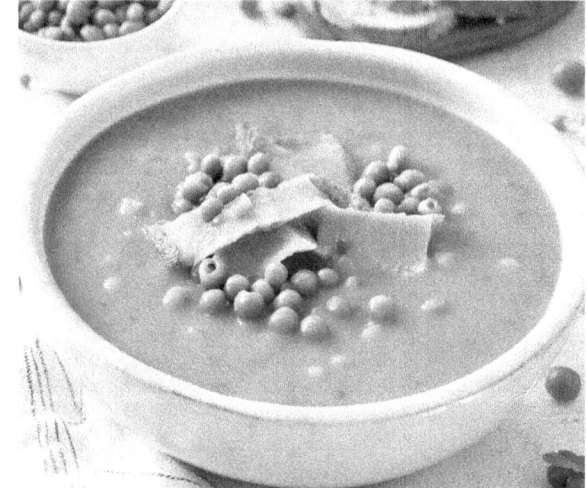

Serves

6

Cooking Time

2 hours

13. Beef Barley Soup

Ingredients

- 1 pound lean beef stew meat, cubed
- 2 tablespoons olive oil
- 1 onion, chopped
- 3 garlic cloves, minced
- 2 carrots, diced
- 2 celery stalks, diced
- 1 cup pearl barley
- 6 cups low-sodium beef broth
- 2 cups water
- 1 teaspoon dried thyme
- 1 teaspoon ground black pepper
- 1/4 cup fresh parsley, chopped (optional, for garnish)

Instructions

1. Heat olive oil in a large pot over medium heat. Add beef and cook until browned, about 5-7 minutes. Remove and set aside.
2. In the same pot, add onion and garlic, cooking for 3-4 minutes until softened.
3. Add carrots and celery, cooking for another 5 minutes.
4. Stir in pearl barley, beef broth, water, dried thyme, and ground black pepper. Return beef to the pot.
5. Bring to a boil, then reduce heat and simmer for 45-50 minutes until barley is tender.
6. Garnish with fresh parsley before serving, if desired.
7. Serve hot.

Nutrition Info per Serving

- Calories: 350
- Carbohydrates: 36g
- Protein: 28g
- Fat: 12g
- Fiber: 8g
- Sodium: 250mg

Serves
6

Cooking Time
1 hour

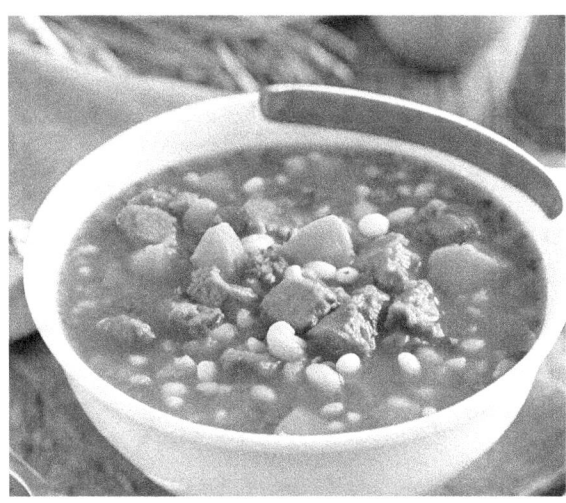

14. Italian Meatball Soup

Ingredients

- 1 pound lean ground turkey or chicken
- 1/4 cup whole wheat breadcrumbs
- 1 egg, beaten
- 2 garlic cloves, minced
- 1 teaspoon dried oregano
- 1 teaspoon ground black pepper
- 2 tablespoons olive oil
- 1 onion, chopped
- 3 garlic cloves, minced
- 1 can (14.5 ounces) diced tomatoes (no salt added)
- 4 cups low-sodium chicken broth
- 2 cups water
- 1 cup whole wheat pasta, such as ditalini or orzo
- 4 cups fresh spinach, chopped
- 1/4 cup grated Parmesan cheese (optional, for garnish)
- 1/4 cup fresh basil, chopped (optional, for garnish)

Instructions

1. In a large bowl, combine ground turkey or chicken, whole wheat breadcrumbs, beaten egg, minced garlic, dried oregano, and ground black pepper. Mix well and form into small meatballs.
2. Heat olive oil in a large pot over medium heat. Add meatballs and cook until browned on all sides, about 5-7 minutes. Remove meatballs and set aside.
3. In the same pot, add onion and garlic, cooking for 3-4 minutes until softened.
4. Stir in diced tomatoes, chicken broth, and water. Bring to a boil.
5. Add whole wheat pasta and cook for 8-10 minutes until pasta is tender.
6. Return meatballs to the pot and stir in chopped spinach. Cook for an additional 5 minutes until spinach is wilted and meatballs are cooked through.
7. Garnish with grated Parmesan cheese and fresh basil before serving, if desired.
8. Serve hot.

Nutrition Info per Serving

- Calories: 300
- Carbohydrates: 28g
- Protein: 28g
- Fat: 10g
- Fiber: 6g
- Sodium: 240mg

Serves

6

Cooking Time

45 minutes

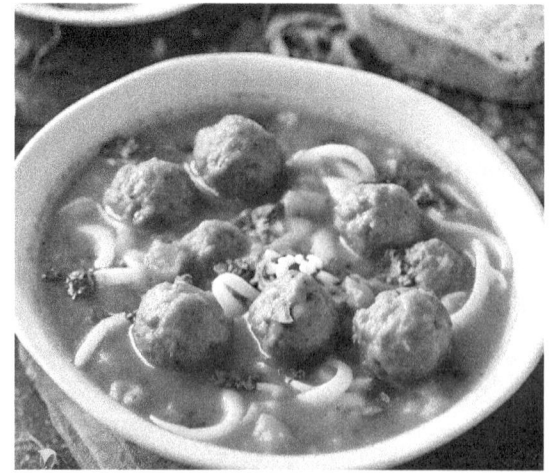

15. Miso Soup with Tofu

Ingredients
- 4 cups low-sodium vegetable broth
- 1/4 cup white miso paste
- 1 block (14 ounces) firm tofu, cubed
- 1 cup baby spinach
- 1 cup sliced mushrooms
- 2 green onions, sliced
- 1 tablespoon grated ginger
- 2 tablespoons low-sodium soy sauce
- 1 sheet nori, cut into small pieces

Instructions
1. In a large pot, bring the vegetable broth to a simmer over medium heat.
2. In a small bowl, mix the miso paste with a small amount of hot broth until smooth, then add it back to the pot.
3. Add the cubed tofu, sliced mushrooms, grated ginger, and soy sauce to the pot. Simmer for 5-7 minutes until the mushrooms are tender.
4. Stir in the baby spinach and nori pieces. Cook for another 2-3 minutes until the spinach is wilted.
5. Serve hot, garnished with sliced green onions.

Nutrition Info per Serving
- Calories: 150
- Carbohydrates: 10g
- Protein: 12g
- Fat: 8g
- Fiber: 2g
- Sodium: 300mg

Serves
4

Cooking Time
15 minutes

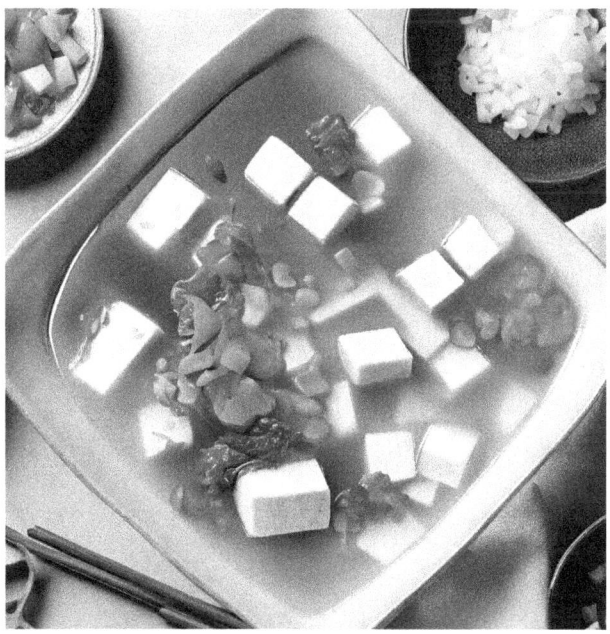

16. Egg Drop Soup

Ingredients

- 4 cups low-sodium chicken broth
- 2 tablespoons low-sodium soy sauce
- 1 tablespoon grated ginger
- 2 eggs, lightly beaten
- 1 cup baby spinach
- 1/2 cup sliced mushrooms
- 2 green onions, sliced
- 1 teaspoon ground black pepper
- 1 teaspoon cornstarch (optional, for thickening)

Instructions

1. In a large pot, bring the chicken broth, soy sauce, and grated ginger to a simmer over medium heat.
2. Add the sliced mushrooms and cook for 5-7 minutes until tender.
3. Stir the cornstarch (if using) into a small amount of cold water, then add it to the pot, stirring constantly until the broth thickens slightly.
4. Slowly pour the beaten eggs into the soup while gently stirring to create ribbons.
5. Add the baby spinach and cook for another 2-3 minutes until wilted.
6. Serve hot, garnished with sliced green onions and ground black pepper.

Nutrition Info per Serving

- Calories: 100
- Carbohydrates: 5g
- Protein: 10g
- Fat: 4g
- Fiber: 1g
- Sodium: 280mg

Serves
4
Cooking Time
15 minutes

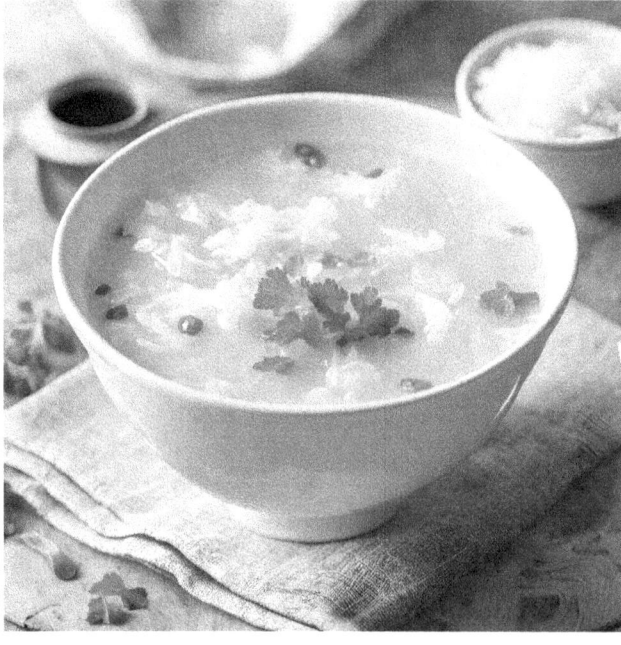

17. Moroccan Chickpea Stew

Ingredients

- 2 tablespoons olive oil
- 1 onion, chopped
- 3 garlic cloves, minced
- 2 carrots, sliced
- 2 celery stalks, sliced
- 1 can (14.5 ounces) diced tomatoes (no salt added)
- 4 cups low-sodium vegetable broth
- 2 cans (15 ounces each) chickpeas, drained and rinsed
- 1 teaspoon ground cumin
- 1 teaspoon ground coriander
- 1 teaspoon ground turmeric
- 1/2 teaspoon ground cinnamon
- 1 teaspoon ground black pepper
- 1/2 cup dried apricots, chopped
- 1/4 cup fresh cilantro, chopped (optional, for garnish)

Instructions

1. Heat olive oil in a large pot over medium heat. Add onion and garlic, cooking for 3-4 minutes until softened.
2. Add carrots and celery, cooking for another 5 minutes.
3. Stir in diced tomatoes, vegetable broth, chickpeas, cumin, coriander, turmeric, cinnamon, and ground black pepper. Bring to a boil, then reduce heat and simmer for 20-25 minutes until vegetables are tender.
4. Stir in the chopped apricots and cook for another 5 minutes.
5. Garnish with fresh cilantro before serving, if desired.
6. Serve hot.

Nutrition Info per Serving

- Calories: 280
- Carbohydrates: 42g
- Protein: 10g
- Fat: 8g
- Fiber: 10g
- Sodium: 240mg

Serves

4

Cooking Time

35 minutes

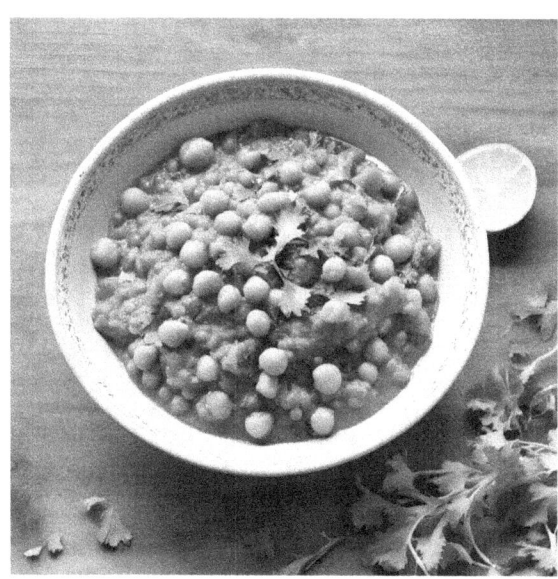

18. Irish Stew with Lamb
Ingredients

- 1 pound lamb stew meat, cubed
- 2 tablespoons olive oil
- 1 onion, chopped
- 3 garlic cloves, minced
- 4 cups low-sodium beef broth
- 2 cups water
- 4 carrots, sliced
- 3 potatoes, peeled and diced
- 2 parsnips, sliced
- 1 teaspoon dried thyme
- 1 teaspoon ground black pepper
- 1/4 cup fresh parsley, chopped (optional, for garnish)

Instructions

1. Heat olive oil in a large pot over medium heat. Add lamb and cook until browned, about 5-7 minutes. Remove and set aside.
2. In the same pot, add onion and garlic, cooking for 3-4 minutes until softened.
3. Return the lamb to the pot and add beef broth, water, carrots, potatoes, parsnips, thyme, and ground black pepper. Bring to a boil, then reduce heat and simmer for 1.5 to 2 hours until the lamb is tender.
4. Garnish with fresh parsley before serving, if desired.
5. Serve hot.

Nutrition Info per Serving

- Calories: 350
- Carbohydrates: 35g
- Protein: 25g
- Fat: 12g
- Fiber: 8g
- Sodium: 280mg

Serves
6
Cooking Time
2 hours

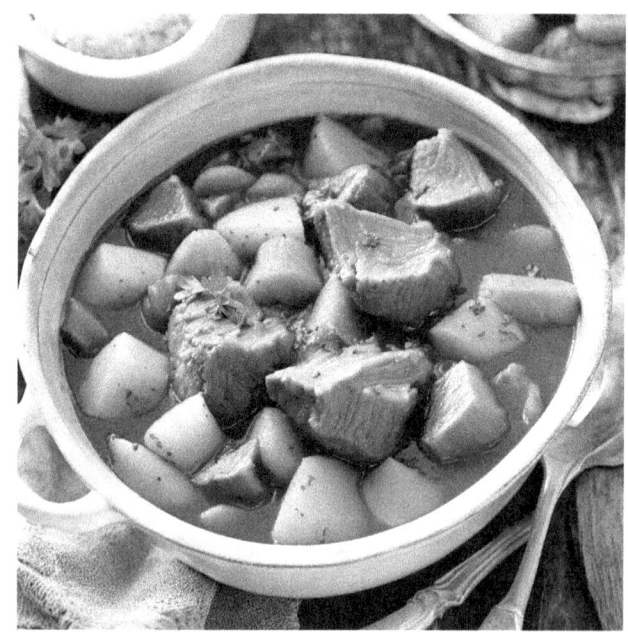

19. Beef and Vegetable Stew

Ingredients

- 1 pound lean beef stew meat, cubed
- 2 tablespoons olive oil
- 1 onion, chopped
- 3 garlic cloves, minced
- 4 cups low-sodium beef broth
- 2 cups water
- 4 carrots, sliced
- 3 potatoes, peeled and diced
- 2 celery stalks, sliced
- 1 cup green beans, trimmed and cut into 1-inch pieces
- 1 teaspoon dried thyme
- 1 teaspoon ground black pepper
- 1/4 cup fresh parsley, chopped (optional, for garnish)

Instructions

1. Heat olive oil in a large pot over medium heat. Add beef and cook until browned, about 5-7 minutes. Remove and set aside.
2. In the same pot, add onion and garlic, cooking for 3-4 minutes until softened.
3. Return the beef to the pot and add beef broth, water, carrots, potatoes, celery, green beans, thyme, and ground black pepper. Bring to a boil, then reduce heat and simmer for 1.5 to 2 hours until the beef and vegetables are tender.
4. Garnish with fresh parsley before serving, if desired.
5. Serve hot.

Nutrition Info per Serving

- Calories: 320
- Carbohydrates: 30g
- Protein: 26g
- Fat: 10g
- Fiber: 7g
- Sodium: 260mg

Serves

6

Cooking Time

2 hours

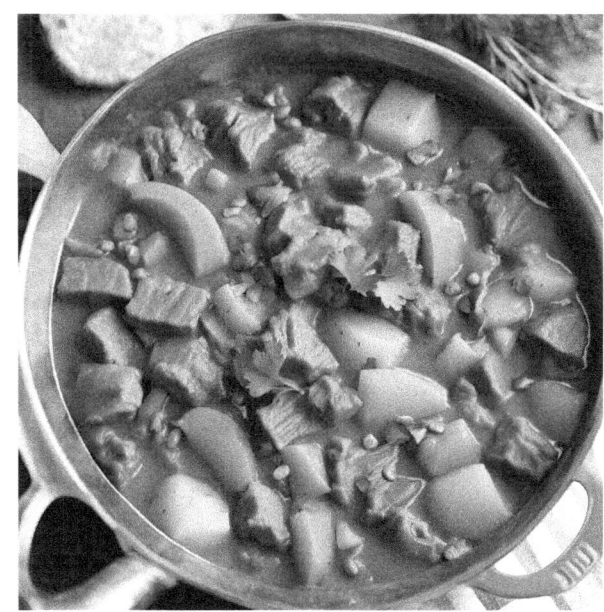

20. Brazilian Black Bean Stew

Ingredients

- 2 tablespoons olive oil
- 1 onion, chopped
- 3 garlic cloves, minced
- 1 red bell pepper, chopped
- 1 green bell pepper, chopped
- 2 cans (15 ounces each) black beans, drained and rinsed
- 4 cups low-sodium vegetable broth
- 1 can (14.5 ounces) diced tomatoes (no salt added)
- 1 teaspoon ground cumin
- 1 teaspoon ground black pepper
- 1/2 teaspoon smoked paprika
- 1/4 cup fresh cilantro, chopped (optional, for garnish)
- 1 lime, cut into wedges (optional, for serving)

Instructions

1. Heat olive oil in a large pot over medium heat. Add onion and garlic, cooking for 3-4 minutes until softened.
2. Add red and green bell peppers, cooking for another 5 minutes.
3. Stir in black beans, vegetable broth, diced tomatoes, ground cumin, ground black pepper, and smoked paprika. Bring to a boil, then reduce heat and simmer for 20-25 minutes.
4. Garnish with fresh cilantro and serve with lime wedges, if desired.
5. Serve hot.

Nutrition Info per Serving

- Calories: 240
- Carbohydrates: 36g
- Protein: 10g
- Fat: 8g
- Fiber: 10g
- Sodium: 220mg

Serves

4

Cooking Time

30 minute

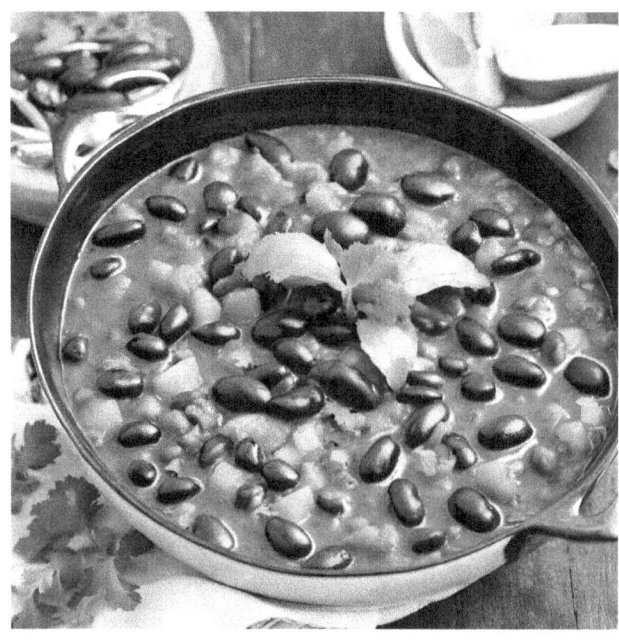

21. Hungarian Mushroom Stew

Ingredients

- 2 tablespoons olive oil
- 1 onion, chopped
- 3 garlic cloves, minced
- 1 pound mushrooms, sliced
- 4 cups low-sodium vegetable broth
- 1 cup unsweetened almond milk
- 1 tablespoon paprika
- 1 teaspoon ground black pepper
- 1/2 cup Greek yogurt (optional, for garnish)
- 1/4 cup fresh dill, chopped (optional, for garnish)

Instructions

1. Heat olive oil in a large pot over medium heat. Add onion and garlic, cooking for 3-4 minutes until softened.
2. Add sliced mushrooms and cook for another 5-7 minutes until tender.
3. Stir in vegetable broth, almond milk, paprika, and ground black pepper. Bring to a boil, then reduce heat and simmer for 15-20 minutes.
4. Garnish with Greek yogurt and fresh dill before serving, if desired.
5. Serve hot.

Nutrition Info per Serving

- Calories: 180
- Carbohydrates: 12g
- Protein: 6g
- Fat: 12g
- Fiber: 3g
- Sodium: 200mg

Serves

4

Cooking Time

30 minutes

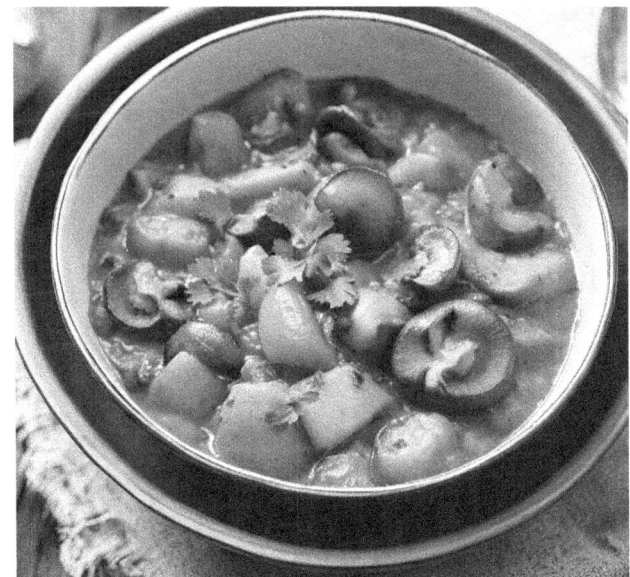

22. Pork and Tomatillo Stew

Ingredients

- 1 pound lean pork shoulder, cubed
- 2 tablespoons olive oil
- 1 onion, chopped
- 3 garlic cloves, minced
- 1 pound tomatillos, husked and chopped
- 1 can (14.5 ounces) diced tomatoes (no salt added)
- 4 cups low-sodium chicken broth
- 1 teaspoon ground cumin
- 1 teaspoon ground black pepper
- 1/4 cup fresh cilantro, chopped (optional, for garnish)

Instructions

1. Heat olive oil in a large pot over medium heat. Add pork and cook until browned, about 5-7 minutes. Remove and set aside.
2. In the same pot, add onion and garlic, cooking for 3-4 minutes until softened.
3. Stir in tomatillos, diced tomatoes, chicken broth, ground cumin, and ground black pepper. Return pork to the pot.
4. Bring to a boil, then reduce heat and simmer for 1.5 to 2 hours until the pork is tender.
5. Garnish with fresh cilantro before serving, if desired.
6. Serve hot.

Nutrition Info per Serving

- Calories: 300
- Carbohydrates: 18g
- Protein: 28g
- Fat: 12g
- Fiber: 5g
- Sodium: 250mg

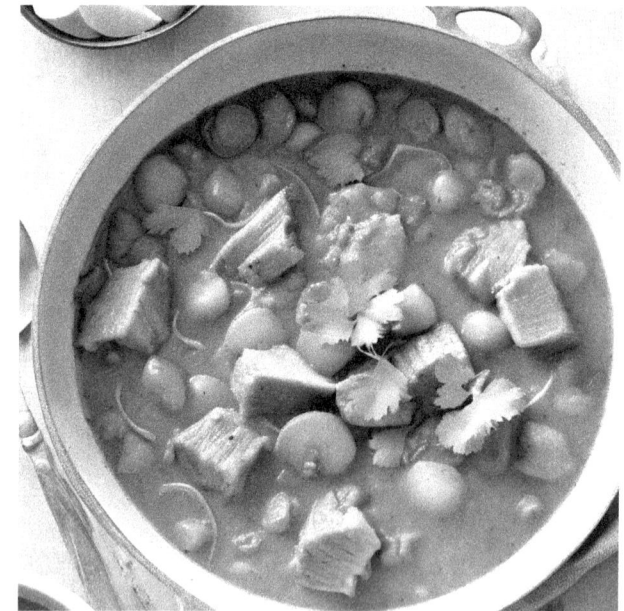

Serves

6

Cooking Time

2 hours

23. Spring Vegetable Soup

Ingredients

- 2 tablespoons olive oil
- 1 onion, chopped
- 3 garlic cloves, minced
- 2 carrots, sliced
- 2 celery stalks, sliced
- 1 zucchini, diced
- 1 cup green beans, trimmed and cut into 1-inch pieces
- 4 cups low-sodium vegetable broth
- 1 cup frozen peas
- 1 teaspoon dried thyme
- 1 teaspoon ground black pepper
- 1/4 cup fresh basil, chopped (optional, for garnish)

Instructions

1. Heat olive oil in a large pot over medium heat. Add onion and garlic, cooking for 3-4 minutes until softened.
2. Add carrots and celery, cooking for another 5 minutes.
3. Stir in zucchini, green beans, vegetable broth, dried thyme, and ground black pepper. Bring to a boil, then reduce heat and simmer for 15-20 minutes until vegetables are tender.
4. Stir in frozen peas and cook for an additional 5 minutes.
5. Garnish with fresh basil before serving, if desired.
6. Serve hot.

Nutrition Info per Serving

- Calories: 150
- Carbohydrates: 24g
- Protein: 4g
- Fat: 5g
- Fiber: 6g
- Sodium: 180mg

Serves

4

Cooking Time

30 minutes

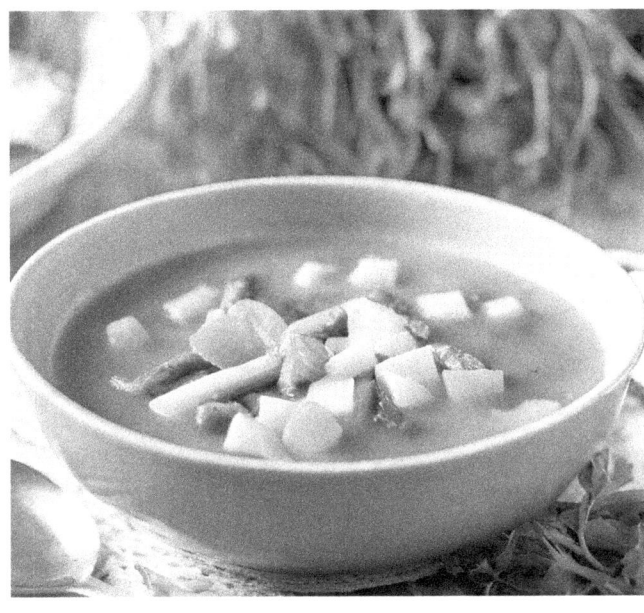

24. Korean Kimchi Stew
Ingredients
- 2 tablespoons olive oil
- 1 onion, chopped
- 3 garlic cloves, minced
- 1 cup kimchi, chopped
- 1 pound tofu, cubed
- 4 cups low-sodium vegetable broth
- 1 tablespoon gochujang (Korean red chili paste)
- 1 teaspoon ground black pepper
- 2 green onions, sliced
- 1/4 cup fresh cilantro, chopped (optional, for garnish)

Instructions
1. Heat olive oil in a large pot over medium heat. Add onion and garlic, cooking for 3-4 minutes until softened.
2. Add chopped kimchi and cook for another 3-4 minutes.
3. Stir in vegetable broth, gochujang, ground black pepper, and tofu. Bring to a boil, then reduce heat and simmer for 15-20 minutes.
4. Garnish with sliced green onions and fresh cilantro before serving, if desired.
5. Serve hot.

Nutrition Info per Serving
- Calories: 180
- Carbohydrates: 10g
- Protein: 12g
- Fat: 12g
- Fiber: 2g
- Sodium: 300mg

Serves
4
Cooking Time
30 minutes

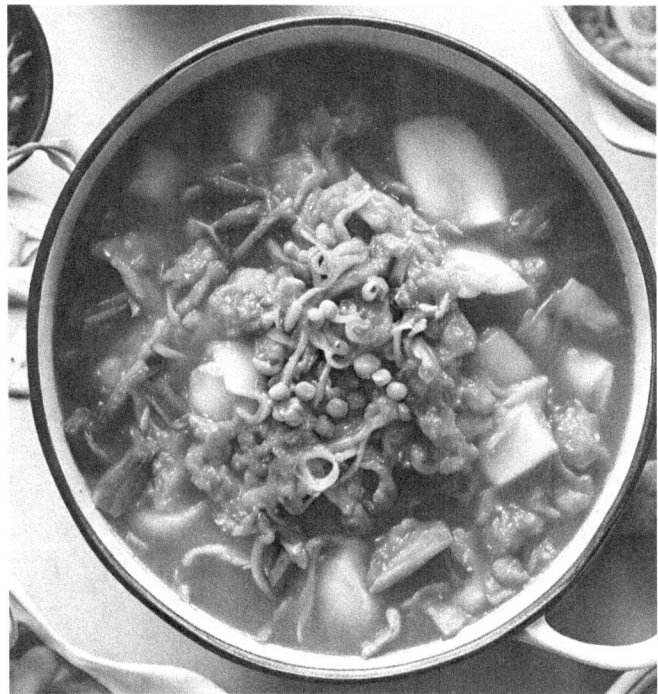

25. Mexican Posole

Ingredients

- 1 pound lean pork shoulder, cubed
- 2 tablespoons olive oil
- 1 onion, chopped
- 3 garlic cloves, minced
- 1 can (14.5 ounces) hominy, drained and rinsed
- 4 cups low-sodium chicken broth
- 1 can (14.5 ounces) diced tomatoes (no salt added)
- 1 tablespoon ground cumin
- 1 teaspoon ground black pepper
- 1 teaspoon dried oregano
- 1/4 cup fresh cilantro, chopped (optional, for garnish)
- 1 lime, cut into wedges (optional, for serving)

Instructions

1. Heat olive oil in a large pot over medium heat. Add pork and cook until browned, about 5-7 minutes. Remove and set aside.
2. In the same pot, add onion and garlic, cooking for 3-4 minutes until softened.
3. Stir in hominy, chicken broth, diced tomatoes, ground cumin, ground black pepper, and dried oregano. Return pork to the pot.
4. Bring to a boil, then reduce heat and simmer for 1.5 to 2 hours until the pork is tender.
5. Garnish with fresh cilantro and serve with lime wedges, if desired.
6. Serve hot.

Nutrition Info per Serving

- Calories: 320
- Carbohydrates: 28g
- Protein: 26g
- Fat: 12g
- Fiber: 6g
- Sodium: 250mg

Serves

6

Cooking Time

2 hours

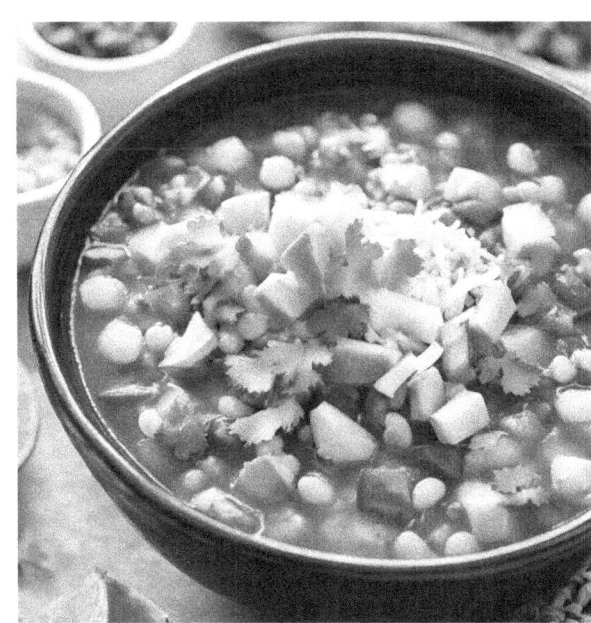

26. Japanese Ramen

Ingredients

- 2 tablespoons olive oil
- 1 onion, chopped
- 3 garlic cloves, minced
- 4 cups low-sodium chicken broth
- 2 cups water
- 1 tablespoon low-sodium soy sauce
- 1 tablespoon miso paste
- 1 teaspoon grated ginger
- 4 ounces shiitake mushrooms, sliced
- 4 cups baby spinach
- 1 package (8 ounces) ramen noodles (without seasoning packet)
- 2 green onions, sliced
- 1 soft-boiled egg per serving (optional, for garnish)

Instructions

1. Heat olive oil in a large pot over medium heat. Add onion and garlic, cooking for 3-4 minutes until softened.
2. Stir in chicken broth, water, soy sauce, miso paste, and grated ginger. Bring to a boil.
3. Add sliced shiitake mushrooms and cook for 5-7 minutes until tender.
4. Add ramen noodles and cook according to package instructions, usually 3-5 minutes.
5. Stir in baby spinach and cook for another 2-3 minutes until wilted.
6. Serve hot, garnished with sliced green onions and a soft-boiled egg, if desired.

Nutrition Info per Serving

- Calories: 250
- Carbohydrates: 35g
- Protein: 10g
- Fat: 8g
- Fiber: 4g
- Sodium: 300mg

Serves

4

Cooking Time

25 minutes

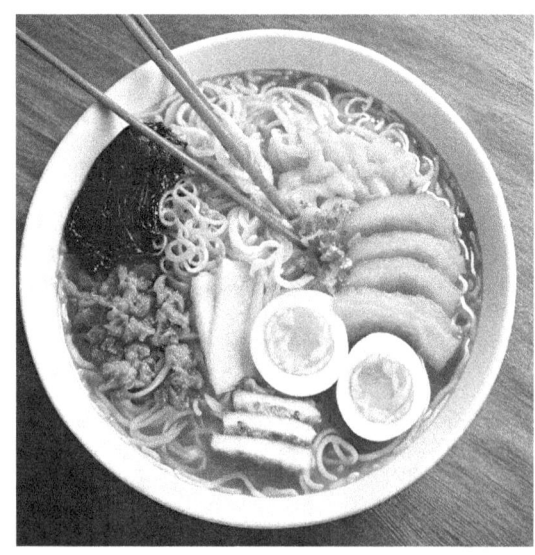

Vegetables

1. Vegetable Lentil Soup
Ingredients
- 2 tablespoons olive oil
- 1 onion, chopped
- 3 garlic cloves, minced
- 2 carrots, diced
- 2 celery stalks, diced
- 1 zucchini, diced
- 1 cup dried lentils, rinsed
- 1 can (14.5 ounces) diced tomatoes (no salt added)
- 6 cups low-sodium vegetable broth
- 1 teaspoon dried thyme
- 1 teaspoon ground cumin
- 1 teaspoon ground black pepper
- 1/4 cup fresh parsley, chopped (optional, for garnish)

Instructions
1. Heat olive oil in a large pot over medium heat. Add onion and garlic, cooking for 3-4 minutes until softened.
2. Add carrots, celery, and zucchini. Cook for another 5 minutes.
3. Stir in lentils, diced tomatoes, vegetable broth, dried thyme, ground cumin, and ground black pepper. Bring to a boil, then reduce heat and simmer for 25-30 minutes until lentils and vegetables are tender.
4. Garnish with fresh parsley before serving, if desired.
5. Serve hot.

Nutrition Info per Serving
- Calories: 220
- Carbohydrates: 35g
- Protein: 10g
- Fat: 6g
- Fiber: 12g
- Sodium: 200mg

Serves
4

Cooking Time
35 minutes

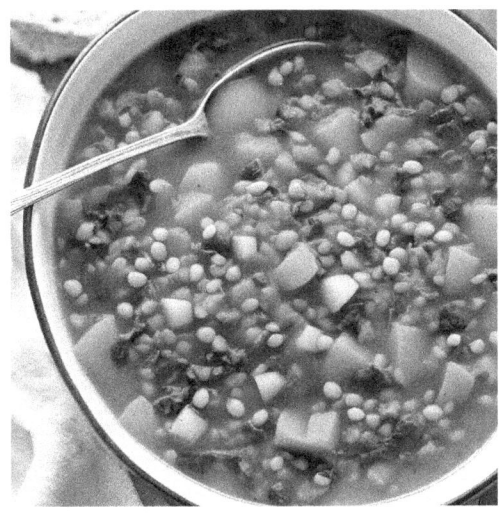

2. Gazpacho

Ingredients

- 4 large tomatoes, chopped
- 1 cucumber, peeled and chopped
- 1 red bell pepper, chopped
- 1 green bell pepper, chopped
- 1 small red onion, chopped
- 2 garlic cloves, minced
- 3 cups tomato juice (low sodium)
- 1/4 cup olive oil
- 2 tablespoons red wine vinegar
- 1 teaspoon ground black pepper
- 1/4 cup fresh basil, chopped (optional, for garnish)

Instructions

1. In a large bowl, combine tomatoes, cucumber, red bell pepper, green bell pepper, red onion, and garlic.
2. Add tomato juice, olive oil, red wine vinegar, and ground black pepper. Stir to combine.
3. Blend the mixture with an immersion blender until smooth, or leave chunky if preferred.
4. Chill in the refrigerator for at least 1 hour before serving.
5. Garnish with fresh basil before serving, if desired.
6. Serve cold.

Nutrition Info per Serving

- Calories: 180
- Carbohydrates: 20g
- Protein: 3g
- Fat: 12g
- Fiber: 4g
- Sodium: 150mg

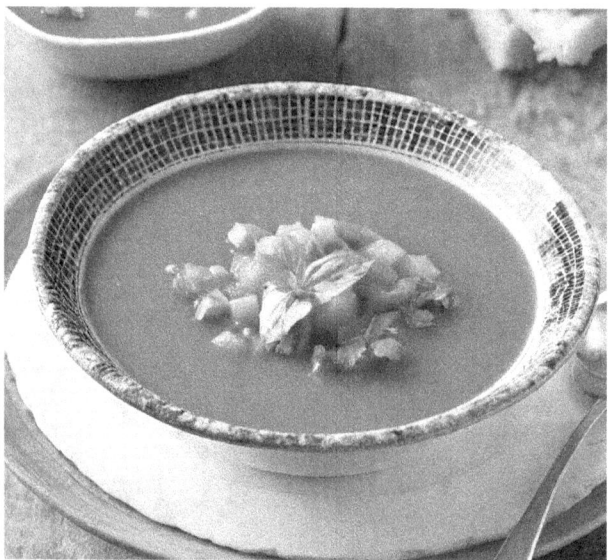

Serves

4

Cooking Time

10 minutes (plus chilling time)

3. Asparagus with Hollandaise Sauce
Ingredients
- 1 pound asparagus, trimmed
- 2 tablespoons olive oil
- 3 egg yolks
- 1 tablespoon fresh lemon juice
- 1/2 cup unsweetened almond milk
- 1 teaspoon ground black pepper

Instructions
1. Preheat oven to 400°F (200°C).
2. Toss asparagus with olive oil and place on a baking sheet. Roast for 15-20 minutes until tender.
3. In a heatproof bowl, whisk together egg yolks and lemon juice until thickened.
4. Place the bowl over a pot of simmering water (double boiler) and slowly whisk in the almond milk until the sauce is thick and creamy.
5. Remove from heat and stir in ground black pepper.
6. Serve the roasted asparagus with the hollandaise sauce drizzled on top.
7. Serve hot.

Nutrition Info per Serving
- Calories: 180
- Carbohydrates: 6g
- Protein: 6g
- Fat: 14g
- Fiber: 3g
- Sodium: 80mg

Serves
4
Cooking Time
20 minutes

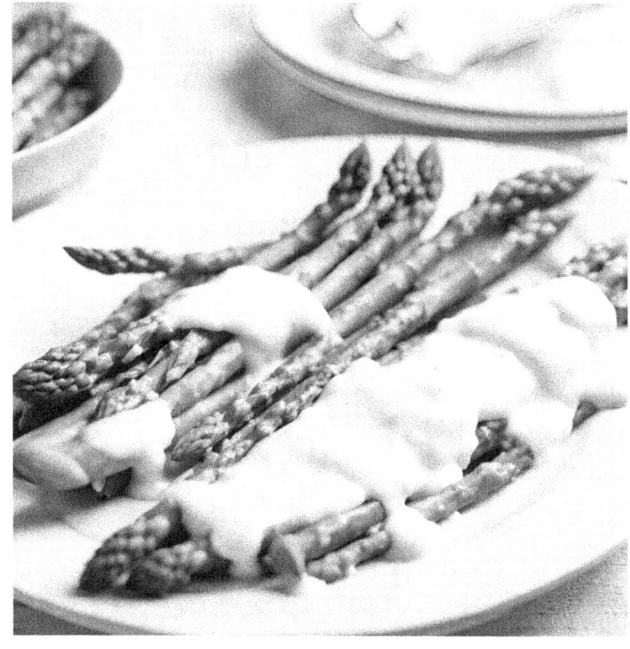

4. Crispy Zucchini Fritters

Ingredients

- 2 medium zucchinis, grated
- 1 teaspoon ground black pepper
- 1/2 cup whole wheat flour
- 2 eggs, beaten
- 1/4 cup green onions, chopped
- 2 tablespoons olive oil

Instructions

1. Place grated zucchini in a colander, sprinkle with ground black pepper, and let sit for 10 minutes to drain excess moisture.
2. In a large bowl, combine grated zucchini, whole wheat flour, beaten eggs, and chopped green onions. Mix well.
3. Heat olive oil in a large skillet over medium heat.
4. Drop spoonfuls of the zucchini mixture into the skillet, flattening them slightly with the back of a spoon.
5. Cook for 3-4 minutes on each side until golden brown and crispy.
6. Drain on paper towels before serving.
7. Serve hot.

Nutrition Info per Serving

- Calories: 160
- Carbohydrates: 14g
- Protein: 6g
- Fat: 10g
- Fiber: 3g
- Sodium: 60mg

Serves

4

Cooking Time

20 minutes

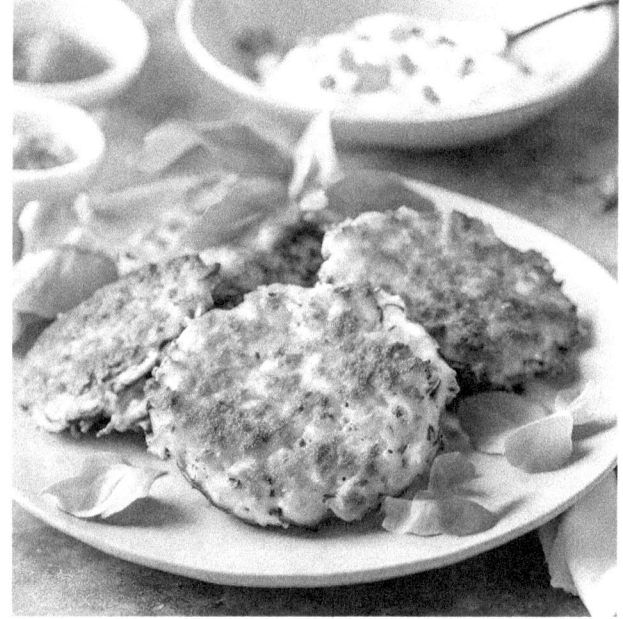

5. Eggplant Dip

Ingredients

- 2 large eggplants
- 2 tablespoons olive oil
- 3 garlic cloves, minced
- 1/4 cup tahini
- 2 tablespoons lemon juice
- 1 teaspoon ground cumin
- 1 teaspoon ground black pepper
- 1/4 cup fresh parsley, chopped (optional, for garnish)

Instructions

1. Preheat oven to 400°F (200°C).
2. Prick the eggplants with a fork and place on a baking sheet. Roast for 40-45 minutes until the skin is charred and the flesh is soft.
3. Let the eggplants cool, then scoop out the flesh into a bowl.
4. Add olive oil, minced garlic, tahini, lemon juice, ground cumin, and ground black pepper to the eggplant. Mix until smooth.
5. Garnish with fresh parsley before serving, if desired.
6. Serve with whole wheat pita bread or vegetable sticks.

Nutrition Info per Serving

- Calories: 120
- Carbohydrates: 12g
- Protein: 3g
- Fat: 8g
- Fiber: 5g
- Sodium: 40mg

Serves

4

Cooking Time

45 minutes

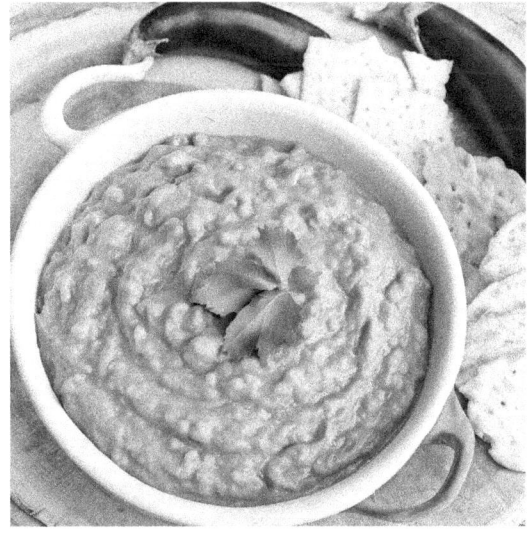

6. Stuffed Mushrooms

Ingredients

- 16 large white mushrooms, stems removed and chopped
- 2 tablespoons olive oil
- 1 small onion, finely chopped
- 3 garlic cloves, minced
- 1/4 cup whole wheat breadcrumbs
- 1/4 cup grated Parmesan cheese
- 2 tablespoons fresh parsley, chopped
- 1 teaspoon ground black pepper

Instructions

1. Preheat oven to 375°F (190°C).
2. Heat olive oil in a skillet over medium heat. Add chopped mushroom stems, onion, and garlic. Cook for 5-7 minutes until tender.
3. Remove from heat and stir in breadcrumbs, Parmesan cheese, parsley, and ground black pepper.
4. Spoon the mixture into the mushroom caps.
5. Place stuffed mushrooms on a baking sheet lined with parchment paper.
6. Bake for 20 minutes until the mushrooms are tender and the tops are golden brown.
7. Serve hot.

Nutrition Info per Serving

- Calories: 120
- Carbohydrates: 10g
- Protein: 5g
- Fat: 7g
- Fiber: 2g
- Sodium: 90mg

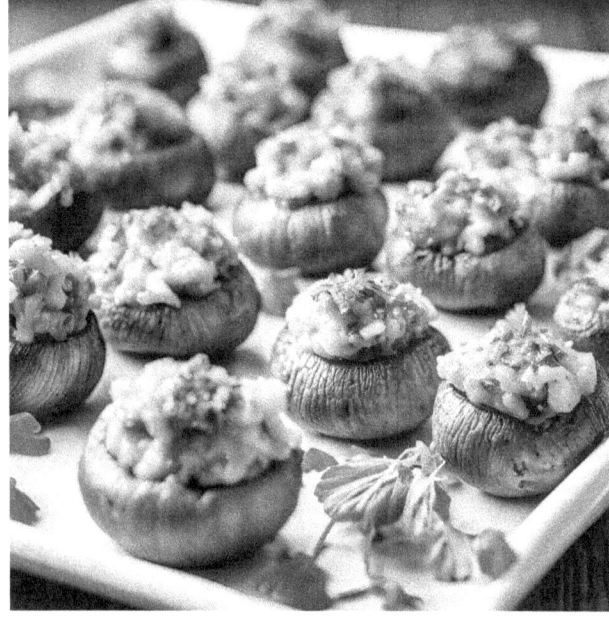

Serves

4

Cooking Time

30 minutes

7. Bruschetta with Tomato and Basil

Ingredients

- 4 ripe tomatoes, diced
- 2 garlic cloves, minced
- 1/4 cup fresh basil, chopped
- 2 tablespoons olive oil
- 1 teaspoon ground black pepper
- 1 whole wheat baguette, sliced

Instructions

1. Preheat oven to 375°F (190°C).
2. In a bowl, combine diced tomatoes, minced garlic, chopped basil, olive oil, and ground black pepper. Mix well.
3. Place baguette slices on a baking sheet and toast in the oven for 5-7 minutes until golden brown.
4. Spoon the tomato mixture onto the toasted baguette slices.
5. Serve immediately.

Nutrition Info per Serving

- Calories: 160
- Carbohydrates: 22g
- Protein: 4g
- Fat: 7g
- Fiber: 3g
- Sodium: 180mg

Serves

4

Cooking Time

10 minutes

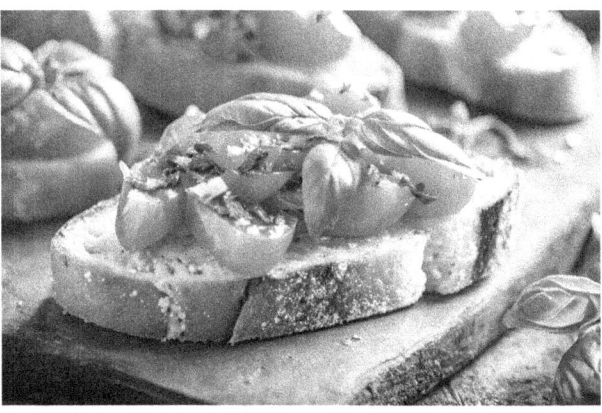

8. Mushroom and Leek Quiche

Ingredients

- 1 whole wheat pie crust
- 2 tablespoons olive oil
- 1 leek, thinly sliced
- 1 cup mushrooms, sliced
- 3 garlic cloves, minced
- 4 eggs
- 1 cup unsweetened almond milk
- 1 teaspoon ground black pepper
- 1/2 cup grated Swiss cheese

Instructions

1. Preheat oven to 375°F (190°C).
2. Heat olive oil in a skillet over medium heat. Add sliced leek, mushrooms, and minced garlic. Cook for 5-7 minutes until tender.
3. In a bowl, whisk together eggs, almond milk, and ground black pepper.
4. Place the cooked vegetables in the pie crust.
5. Pour the egg mixture over the vegetables.
6. Sprinkle with grated Swiss cheese.
7. Bake for 35-40 minutes until the quiche is set and golden brown.
8. Let cool slightly before serving.
9. Serve warm.

Nutrition Info per Serving

- Calories: 250
- Carbohydrates: 18g
- Protein: 10g
- Fat: 16g
- Fiber: 3g
- Sodium: 200mg

Serves
6

Cooking Time
45 minutes

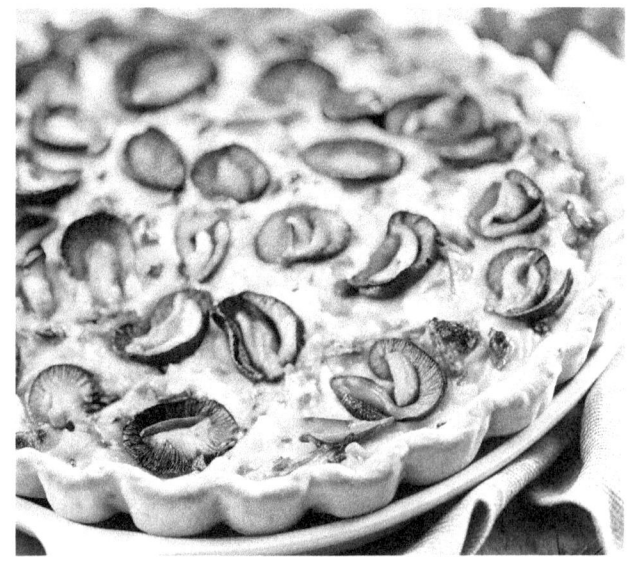

9. Vegetable Stir Fry with Tofu

Ingredients

- 1 block (14 ounces) firm tofu, cubed
- 2 tablespoons olive oil
- 1 onion, sliced
- 2 garlic cloves, minced
- 1 red bell pepper, sliced
- 1 yellow bell pepper, sliced
- 1 zucchini, sliced
- 1 cup broccoli florets
- 1 cup snap peas
- 2 tablespoons low-sodium soy sauce
- 1 tablespoon rice vinegar
- 1 teaspoon ground black pepper
- 1/4 cup fresh cilantro, chopped (optional, for garnish)

Instructions

1. Heat 1 tablespoon of olive oil in a large skillet or wok over medium-high heat. Add cubed tofu and cook until golden brown on all sides, about 5-7 minutes. Remove from the skillet and set aside.
2. In the same skillet, heat the remaining olive oil. Add onion and garlic, cooking for 3-4 minutes until softened.
3. Add red and yellow bell peppers, zucchini, broccoli, and snap peas. Stir-fry for 5-7 minutes until vegetables are tender-crisp.
4. Return tofu to the skillet and stir in soy sauce, rice vinegar, and ground black pepper. Cook for another 2-3 minutes until heated through.
5. Garnish with fresh cilantro before serving, if desired.
6. Serve hot.

Nutrition Info per Serving

- Calories: 220
- Carbohydrates: 14g
- Protein: 12g
- Fat: 14g
- Fiber: 4g
- Sodium: 300mg

Serves

4

Cooking Time

20 minutes

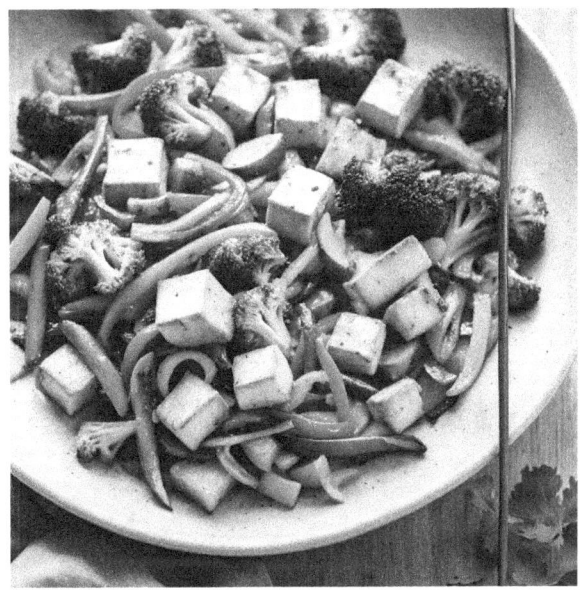

10. Grilled Asparagus with Lemon Tarragon Dressing

Ingredients

- 1 pound asparagus, trimmed
- 2 tablespoons olive oil
- 1 lemon, juiced and zested
- 1 tablespoon fresh tarragon, chopped
- 1 teaspoon ground black pepper

Instructions

1. Preheat grill to medium-high heat.
2. Toss asparagus with 1 tablespoon of olive oil and ground black pepper.
3. Grill asparagus for 5-7 minutes, turning occasionally until tender and slightly charred.
4. In a small bowl, whisk together lemon juice, lemon zest, remaining olive oil, and chopped tarragon.
5. Drizzle the lemon tarragon dressing over the grilled asparagus.
6. Serve hot.

Nutrition Info per Serving

- Calories: 110
- Carbohydrates: 7g
- Protein: 3g
- Fat: 9g
- Fiber: 3g
- Sodium: 20mg

Serves
4
Cooking Time
10 minutes

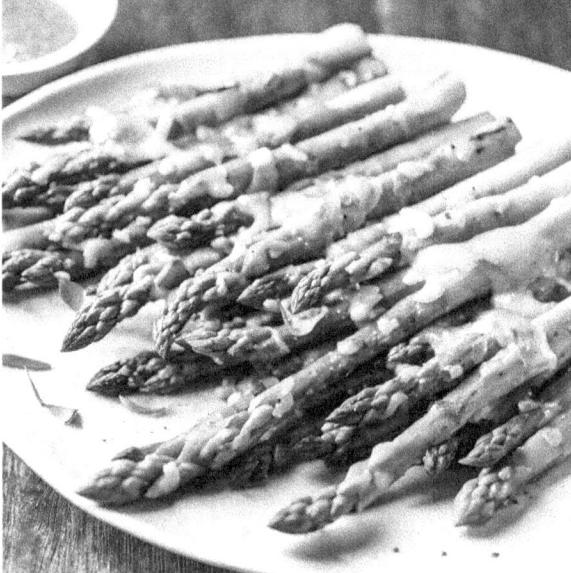

11. Spaghetti Squash with Tomato Sauce

Ingredients

- 1 large spaghetti squash
- 2 tablespoons olive oil
- 1 onion, chopped
- 3 garlic cloves, minced
- 1 can (14.5 ounces) diced tomatoes (no salt added)
- 1 teaspoon dried oregano
- 1 teaspoon ground black pepper
- 1/4 cup fresh basil, chopped

Instructions

1. Preheat oven to 375°F (190°C).
2. Cut the spaghetti squash in half lengthwise and remove the seeds. Drizzle with 1 tablespoon of olive oil.
3. Place the squash halves cut side down on a baking sheet lined with parchment paper. Bake for 35-40 minutes until tender.
4. While the squash is baking, heat the remaining olive oil in a large skillet over medium heat. Add onion and garlic, cooking for 3-4 minutes until softened.
5. Stir in diced tomatoes, dried oregano, and ground black pepper. Simmer for 15-20 minutes until the sauce thickens.
6. Once the squash is done, use a fork to scrape out the strands of squash into a large bowl.
7. Serve the spaghetti squash topped with the tomato sauce and garnished with fresh basil.
8. Serve hot.

Nutrition Info per Serving

- Calories: 140
- Carbohydrates: 22g
- Protein: 3g
- Fat: 7g
- Fiber: 4g
- Sodium: 100mg

Serves

4

Cooking Time

40 minutes

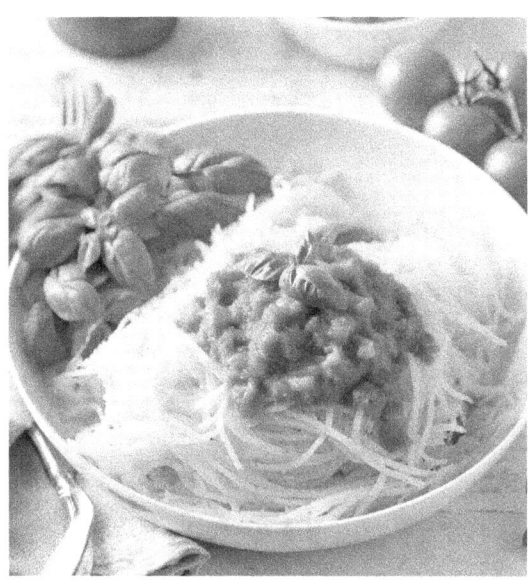

12. Sweet Potato and Black Bean Chili

Ingredients

- 2 tablespoons olive oil
- 1 onion, chopped
- 3 garlic cloves, minced
- 2 medium sweet potatoes, peeled and diced
- 1 red bell pepper, chopped
- 1 can (15 ounces) black beans, drained and rinsed
- 1 can (14.5 ounces) diced tomatoes (no salt added)
- 4 cups low-sodium vegetable broth
- 1 tablespoon chili powder
- 1 teaspoon ground cumin
- 1 teaspoon ground black pepper
- 1/4 cup fresh cilantro, chopped (optional, for garnish)

Instructions

1. Heat olive oil in a large pot over medium heat. Add onion and garlic, cooking for 3-4 minutes until softened.
2. Add diced sweet potatoes and red bell pepper, cooking for another 5 minutes.
3. Stir in black beans, diced tomatoes, vegetable broth, chili powder, ground cumin, and ground black pepper. Bring to a boil, then reduce heat and simmer for 25-30 minutes until sweet potatoes are tender.
4. Garnish with fresh cilantro before serving, if desired.
5. Serve hot.

Nutrition Info per Serving

- Calories: 220
- Carbohydrates: 40g
- Protein: 6g
- Fat: 6g
- Fiber: 10g
- Sodium: 220mg

Serves

4

Cooking Time

35 minutes

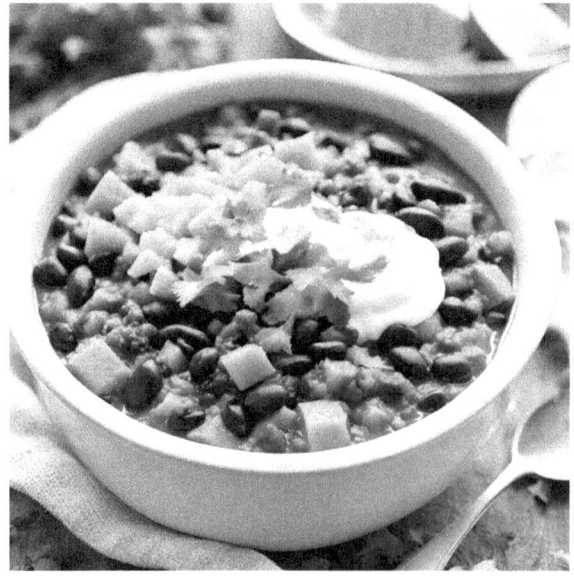

13. Zucchini Noodle Salad

Ingredients

- 4 medium zucchinis, spiralized into noodles
- 1 cup cherry tomatoes, halved
- 1/2 red onion, thinly sliced
- 1/4 cup fresh basil, chopped
- 1/4 cup fresh parsley, chopped
- 2 tablespoons olive oil
- 1 tablespoon balsamic vinegar
- 1 teaspoon ground black pepper

Instructions

1. In a large bowl, combine zucchini noodles, cherry tomatoes, red onion, basil, and parsley.
2. In a small bowl, whisk together olive oil, balsamic vinegar, and ground black pepper.
3. Pour the dressing over the salad and toss to combine.
4. Serve immediately.

Nutrition Info per Serving

- Calories: 120
- Carbohydrates: 10g
- Protein: 3g
- Fat: 9g
- Fiber: 3g
- Sodium: 20mg

Serves

4

Cooking Time

10 minutes

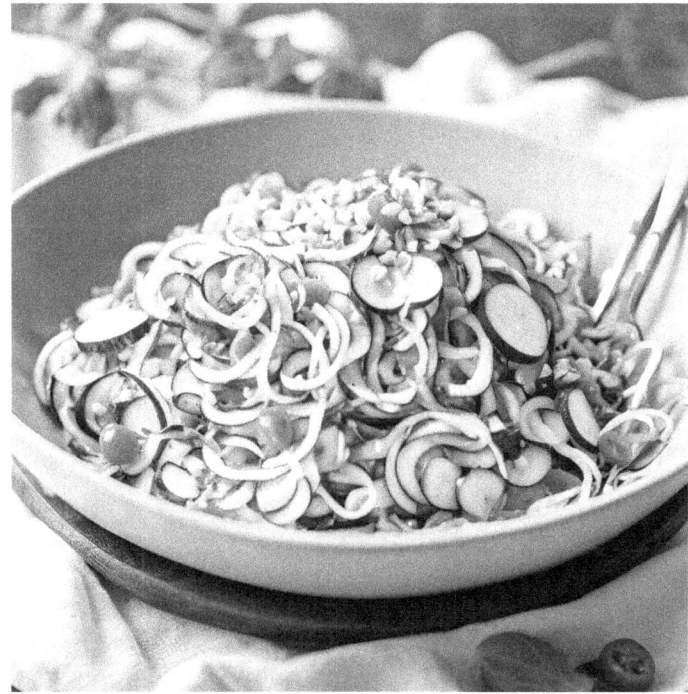

10-WEEK MEAL PLAN

Week 1
Monday:
- Breakfast: Apple Cinnamon Oatmeal
- Lunch: Poached Chicken Salad
- Dinner: Grilled Salmon with Dill
- Snack: Fresh fruit (apple, orange)

Tuesday:
- Breakfast: Banana Nut Oatmeal
- Lunch: Vegetable Lentil Soup
- Dinner: Chicken and Vegetable Stir-Fry
- Snack: Greek Yogurt with Mixed Nuts and Honey

Wednesday:
- Breakfast: Berry Oatmeal Smoothie
- Lunch: Miso Soup with Tofu
- Dinner: Baked Cod with Lemon and Capers
- Snack: Carrot sticks with hummus

Thursday:
- Breakfast: Vegetable Frittata
- Lunch: Gazpacho
- Dinner: Tilapia Piccata
- Snack: Mixed berries

Friday:
- Breakfast: Spinach and Mushroom Omelette
- Lunch: Greek Salad with Grilled Chicken
- Dinner: Herb-Crusted Halibut
- Snack: Whole wheat crackers with avocado

Saturday:
- Breakfast: Kale and Spinach Smoothie
- Lunch: Bruschetta with Tomato and Basil
- Dinner: Grilled Lemon Herb Chicken
- Snack: Sliced cucumber with tzatziki

Sunday:
- Breakfast: Berry Beet Smoothie
- Lunch: Quinoa Breakfast Bowl
- Dinner: Roasted Butternut Squash Soup
- Snack: Almonds

Week 2

Monday:
- Breakfast: Greek Yogurt with Mixed Nuts and Honey
- Lunch: Spaghetti Squash with Tomato Sauce
- Dinner: Smoked Haddock Chowder
- Snack: Fresh fruit (apple, orange)

Tuesday:
- Breakfast: Pineapple Turmeric Smoothie
- Lunch: Caprese Salad with an Egg
- Dinner: Chicken Paella with Brown Rice
- Snack: Carrot sticks with hummus

Wednesday:
- Breakfast: Berry Parfait
- Lunch: Stuffed Mushrooms
- Dinner: Grilled Sea Bass with Mango Salsa
- Snack: Mixed berries

Thursday:
- Breakfast: Quinoa Breakfast Bowl
- Lunch: Chicken and Vegetable Stir-Fry
- Dinner: Chicken Noodle Soup
- Snack: Greek Yogurt with Mixed Nuts and Honey

Friday:
- Breakfast: Whole Wheat Pancakes
- Lunch: Cabbage Detox Soup
- Dinner: Shrimp Stir-Fry with Vegetables
- Snack: Whole wheat crackers with avocado

Saturday:
- Breakfast: Barley Porridge
- Lunch: Eggplant Dip with whole wheat pita
- Dinner: Poached Salmon with Asparagus
- Snack: Sliced cucumber with tzatziki

Sunday:
- Breakfast: Whole Grain Waffles
- Lunch: Asparagus with Hollandaise Sauce
- Dinner: Sweet Potato and Black Bean Chili
- Snack: Almonds

Week 3

Monday:
- Breakfast: Turkey and Spinach Breakfast Sausages
- Lunch: Spring Vegetable Soup
- Dinner: Grilled Lemon Herb Chicken
- Snack: Fresh fruit (apple, orange)

Tuesday:
- Breakfast: Rice Porridge with Berries
- Lunch: Beetroot and Ginger Soup
- Dinner: Turkey and White Bean Chili
- Snack: Greek Yogurt with Mixed Nuts and Honey

Wednesday:
- Breakfast: Sweet Potato Congee
- Lunch: Miso Soup with Tofu
- Dinner: Beef and Vegetable Stew
- Snack: Carrot sticks with hummus

Thursday:
- Breakfast: Millet Porridge with Apples and Cinnamon
- Lunch: Mushroom and Leek Quiche
- Dinner: Grilled Asparagus with Lemon Tarragon Dressing
- Snack: Mixed berries

Friday:
- Breakfast: Buckwheat Porridge with Honey and Walnuts
- Lunch: Chicken and Turkey Meatballs
- Dinner: Pork and Tomatillo Stew
- Snack: Whole wheat crackers with avocado

Saturday:
- Breakfast: Caprese Salad with an Egg
- Lunch: Egg Drop Soup
- Dinner: Seafood Paella
- Snack: Sliced cucumber with tzatziki

Sunday:
- Breakfast: Watermelon Salad with Mint and Feta
- Lunch: Turkey Bolognese
- Dinner: Moroccan Chickpea Stew
- Snack: Almonds

Week 4

Monday:
- Breakfast: Nutty Granola
- Lunch: Vegetable Lentil Soup
- Dinner: Grilled Salmon with Dill
- Snack: Fresh fruit (apple, orange)

Tuesday:
- Breakfast: Seed Mix Topped Yogurt
- Lunch: Gazpacho
- Dinner: Chicken Cacciatore
- Snack: Greek Yogurt with Mixed Nuts and Honey

Wednesday:
- Breakfast: Coconut and Almond Chia Breakfast Bowl
- Lunch: Bruschetta with Tomato and Basil
- Dinner: Fisherman's Stew
- Snack: Carrot sticks with hummus

Thursday:
- Breakfast: Whole Wheat Pancakes
- Lunch: Chicken Paella with Brown Rice
- Dinner: Tilapia Piccata
- Snack: Mixed berries

Friday:
- Breakfast: Barley Porridge
- Lunch: Stuffed Mushrooms
- Dinner: Smoked Haddock Chowder
- Snack: Whole wheat crackers with avocado

Saturday:
- Breakfast: Quinoa Breakfast Bowl
- Lunch: Asparagus with Hollandaise Sauce
- Dinner: Grilled Lemon Herb Chicken
- Snack: Sliced cucumber with tzatziki

Sunday:
- Breakfast: Spinach and Mushroom Omelette
- Lunch: Spring Vegetable Soup
- Dinner: Sweet Potato and Black Bean Chili
- Snack: Almonds

Week 5

Monday:
- Breakfast: Apple Cinnamon Oatmeal
- Lunch: Mushroom and Leek Quiche
- Dinner: Seafood Paella
- Snack: Fresh fruit (apple, orange)

Tuesday:
- Breakfast: Pineapple Turmeric Smoothie
- Lunch: Beetroot and Ginger Soup
- Dinner: Chicken Noodle Soup
- Snack: Greek Yogurt with Mixed Nuts and Honey

Wednesday:
- Breakfast: Berry Parfait
- Lunch: Turkey and White Bean Chili
- Dinner: Herb-Crusted Halibut
- Snack: Carrot sticks with hummus

Thursday:
- Breakfast: Coconut and Almond Chia Breakfast Bowl
- Lunch: Eggplant Dip with whole wheat pita
- Dinner: Spicy Sweet Potato Soup
- Snack: Mixed berries

Friday:
- Breakfast: Barley Porridge
- Lunch: Mushroom and Leek Quiche
- Dinner: Tilapia Piccata
- Snack: Whole wheat crackers with avocado

Saturday:
- Breakfast: Whole Grain Waffles
- Lunch: Vegetable Lentil Soup
- Dinner: Poached Salmon with Asparagus
- Snack: Sliced cucumber with tzatziki

Sunday:
- Breakfast: Nutty Granola
- Lunch: Gazpacho
- Dinner: Beef and Vegetable Stew
- Snack: Almonds

Week 6

Monday:
- Breakfast: Quinoa Breakfast Bowl
- Lunch: Turkey Bolognese
- Dinner: Grilled Sea Bass with Mango Salsa
- Snack: Fresh fruit (apple, orange)

Tuesday:
- Breakfast: Millet Porridge with Apples and Cinnamon
- Lunch: Greek Salad with Grilled Chicken
- Dinner: Smoked Turkey Breast
- Snack: Greek Yogurt with Mixed Nuts and Honey

Wednesday:
- Breakfast: Spinach and Mushroom Omelette
- Lunch: Chicken Paella with Brown Rice
- Dinner: Mackerel with Tomato Salad
- Snack: Carrot sticks with hummus

Thursday:
- Breakfast: Barley Porridge
- Lunch: Cabbage Detox Soup
- Dinner: Turkey Meatloaf
- Snack: Mixed berries

Friday:
- Breakfast: Pineapple Turmeric Smoothie
- Lunch: Bruschetta with Tomato and Basil
- Dinner: Lemon Butter Scampi
- Snack: Whole wheat crackers with avocado

Saturday:
- Breakfast: Zucchini Noodle Salad
- Lunch: Eggplant Dip with whole wheat pita
- Dinner: Grilled Asparagus with Lemon Tarragon Dressing
- Snack: Sliced cucumber with tzatziki

Sunday:
- Breakfast: Seed Mix Topped Yogurt
- Lunch: Spring Vegetable Soup
- Dinner: Pork and Tomatillo Stew
- Snack: Almonds

Week 7

Monday:
- Breakfast: Buckwheat Porridge with Honey and Walnuts
- Lunch: Vegetable Lentil Soup
- Dinner: Chicken Cacciatore
- Snack: Fresh fruit (apple, orange)

Tuesday:
- Breakfast: Coconut and Almond Chia Breakfast Bowl
- Lunch: Miso Soup with Tofu
- Dinner: Grilled Lemon Herb Chicken
- Snack: Greek Yogurt with Mixed Nuts and Honey

Wednesday:
- Breakfast: Whole Grain Waffles
- Lunch: Chicken and Vegetable Stir-Fry
- Dinner: Baked Trout with Walnut Crust
- Snack: Carrot sticks with hummus

Thursday:
- Breakfast: Nutty Granola
- Lunch: Sweet Potato and Black Bean Chili
- Dinner: Shrimp Stir-Fry with Vegetables
- Snack: Mixed berries

Friday:
- Breakfast: Rice Porridge with Berries
- Lunch: Bruschetta with Tomato and Basil
- Dinner: Beef Barley Soup
- Snack: Whole wheat crackers with avocado

Saturday:
- Breakfast: Caprese Salad with an Egg
- Lunch: Turkey and Spinach Meatballs
- Dinner: Spicy Tuna Poke Bowl
- Snack: Sliced cucumber with tzatziki

Sunday:
- Breakfast: Spinach and Mushroom Omelette
- Lunch: Egg Drop Soup
- Dinner: Moroccan Chickpea Stew
- Snack: Almonds

Week 8

Monday:
- Breakfast: Greek Yogurt with Mixed Nuts and Honey
- Lunch: Mushroom and Leek Quiche
- Dinner: Fisherman's Stew
- Snack: Fresh fruit (apple, orange)

Tuesday:
- Breakfast: Berry Parfait
- Lunch: Gazpacho
- Dinner: Chicken and Turkey Sausage Jambalaya
- Snack: Greek Yogurt with Mixed Nuts and Honey

Wednesday:
- Breakfast: Kale and Spinach Smoothie
- Lunch: Stuffed Mushrooms
- Dinner: Seafood and Spinach Lasagna
- Snack: Carrot sticks with hummus

Thursday:
- Breakfast: Sweet Potato Congee
- Lunch: Asparagus with Hollandaise Sauce
- Dinner: Tilapia Piccata
- Snack: Mixed berries

Friday:
- Breakfast: Millet Porridge with Apples and Cinnamon
- Lunch: Miso Soup with Tofu
- Dinner: Pork and Tomatillo Stew
- Snack: Whole wheat crackers with avocado

Saturday:
- Breakfast: Watermelon Salad with Mint and Feta
- Lunch: Chicken Noodle Soup
- Dinner: Spaghetti Squash with Tomato Sauce
- Snack: Sliced cucumber with tzatziki

Sunday:
- Breakfast: Apple Cinnamon Oatmeal
- Lunch: Spring Vegetable Soup
- Dinner: Beef and Vegetable Stew
- Snack: Almonds

Week 9
Monday:
- Breakfast: Barley Porridge
- Lunch: Chicken Paella with Brown Rice
- Dinner: Grilled Salmon with Dill
- Snack: Fresh fruit (apple, orange)

Tuesday:
- Breakfast: Zucchini Noodle Salad
- Lunch: Eggplant Dip with whole wheat pita
- Dinner: Chicken and Vegetable Stir-Fry
- Snack: Greek Yogurt with Mixed Nuts and Honey

Wednesday:
- Breakfast: Buckwheat Porridge with Honey and Walnuts
- Lunch: Gazpacho
- Dinner: Baked Cod with Lemon and Capers
- Snack: Carrot sticks with hummus

Thursday:
- Breakfast: Nutty Granola
- Lunch: Greek Salad with Grilled Chicken
- Dinner: Fisherman's Stew
- Snack: Mixed berries

Friday:
- Breakfast: Seed Mix Topped Yogurt
- Lunch: Bruschetta with Tomato and Basil
- Dinner: Chicken Cacciatore
- Snack: Whole wheat crackers with avocado

Saturday:
- Breakfast: Pineapple Turmeric Smoothie
- Lunch: Miso Soup with Tofu
- Dinner: Grilled Sea Bass with Mango Salsa
- Snack: Sliced cucumber with tzatziki

Sunday:
- Breakfast: Whole Wheat Pancakes
- Lunch: Sweet Potato and Black Bean Chili
- Dinner: Smoked Haddock Chowder
- Snack: Almonds

Week 10

Monday:
- Breakfast: Millet Porridge with Apples and Cinnamon
- Lunch: Spring Vegetable Soup
- Dinner: Seafood Paella
- Snack: Fresh fruit (apple, orange)

Tuesday:
- Breakfast: Spinach and Mushroom Omelette
- Lunch: Egg Drop Soup
- Dinner: Grilled Asparagus with Lemon Tarragon Dressing
- Snack: Greek Yogurt with Mixed Nuts and Honey

Wednesday:
- Breakfast: Coconut and Almond Chia Breakfast Bowl
- Lunch: Bruschetta with Tomato and Basil
- Dinner: Chicken Noodle Soup
- Snack: Carrot sticks with hummus

Thursday:
- Breakfast: Berry Parfait
- Lunch: Chicken and Turkey Meatballs
- Dinner: Spicy Sweet Potato Soup
- Snack: Mixed berries

Friday:
- Breakfast: Kale and Spinach Smoothie
- Lunch: Stuffed Mushrooms
- Dinner: Grilled Lemon Herb Chicken
- Snack: Whole wheat crackers with avocado

Saturday:
- Breakfast: Greek Yogurt with Mixed Nuts and Honey
- Lunch: Vegetable Lentil Soup
- Dinner: Pork and Tomatillo Stew
- Snack: Sliced cucumber with tzatziki

Sunday:
- Breakfast: Apple Cinnamon Oatmeal
- Lunch: Miso Soup with Tofu
- Dinner: Moroccan Chickpea Stew
- Snack: Almonds

Weekly Meal planner+ Journal

	BREAKFAST	LUNCH	DINNER	SNACKS
MON				
TUE				
WED				
THU				
FRI				
SAT				
SUN				

What are your typical daily meals and snacks like? How often do you consume foods high in sodium or saturated fats?

....

....

....

....

....

....

....

Weekly Meal planner+ Journal

	BREAKFAST	LUNCH	DINNER	SNACKS
MON				
TUE				
WED				
THU				
FRI				
SAT				
SUN				

Can you recall any specific foods or drinks that seem to trigger your AFib episodes? How do you feel after consuming caffeine or alcohol?

....

....

....

....

....

....

....

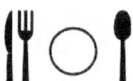

Weekly Meal planner+ Journal

	BREAKFAST	LUNCH	DINNER	SNACKS
MON				
TUE				
WED				
THU				
FRI				
SAT				
SUN				

Do you pay attention to portion sizes when you eat? What strategies could you use to control portion sizes effectively?

....

....

....

....

....

....

....

Weekly Meal planner+ Journal

	BREAKFAST	LUNCH	DINNER	SNACKS
MON				
TUE				
WED				
THU				
FRI				
SAT				
SUN				

What are some ways you can incorporate more fruits and vegetables into your meals? How can you include more whole grains in your diet?

....

....

....

....

....

....

....

Weekly Meal planner+ Journal

	BREAKFAST	LUNCH	DINNER	SNACKS
MON				
TUE				
WED				
THU				
FRI				
SAT				
SUN				

What are your short-term and long-term goals for modifying your diet to manage AFib? How will you track your progress towards these goals?

....

....

....

....

....

....

....

Weekly Meal planner+ Journal

	BREAKFAST	LUNCH	DINNER	SNACKS
MON				
TUE				
WED				
THU				
FRI				
SAT				
SUN				

Do you know how to read food labels to identify sodium and sugar content? What information on food labels will you pay close attention to?

....

....

....

....

....

....

Weekly Meal planner+ Journal

	BREAKFAST	LUNCH	DINNER	SNACKS
MON				
TUE				
WED				
THU				
FRI				
SAT				
SUN				

Have you discussed with your doctor the use of supplements or vitamins that may benefit heart health How do you currently ensure you are getting essential nutrients in your diet?

....

....

....

....

....

....

....

Weekly Meal planner+ Journal

	BREAKFAST	LUNCH	DINNER	SNACKS
MON				
TUE				
WED				
THU				
FRI				
SAT				
SUN				

Who can support you in making dietary changes to manage your AFib? How can your family and friends help you stay motivated?

....

....

....

....

....

....

....

Weekly Meal planner+ Journal

	BREAKFAST	LUNCH	DINNER	SNACKS
MON				
TUE				
WED				
THU				
FRI				
SAT				
SUN				

What milestones will you celebrate along your journey to a healthier diet? How will you stay motivated if you face challenges or setbacks?

....

....

....

....

....

....

....

Weekly Meal planner+ Journal

	BREAKFAST	LUNCH	DINNER	SNACKS
MON				
TUE				
WED				
THU				
FRI				
SAT				
SUN				

How do you envision your diet evolving over the next year to better manage your AFib? What strategies will you implement to maintain a heart-healthy diet in the long term?

....

....

....

....

....

....

....

Scan the QR code below to get a surprise bonus